THE
FORAGER'S
ALMANAC

This book is for you, Mum.
May you rest among the wildflowers.

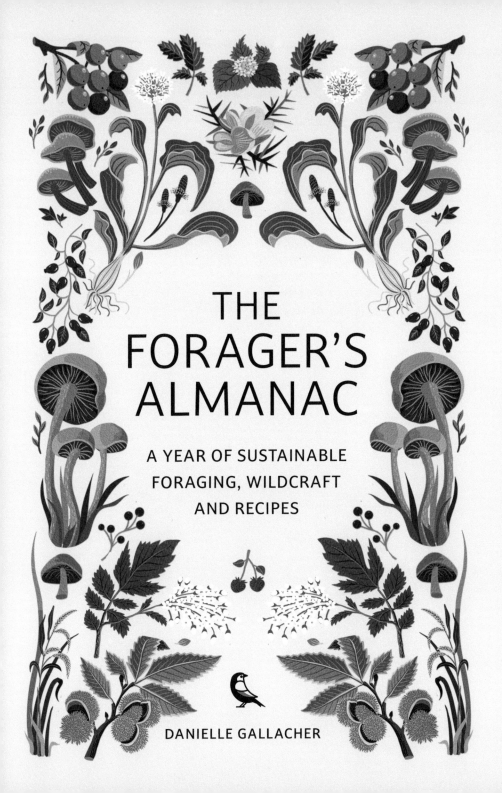

THE FORAGER'S ALMANAC

A YEAR OF SUSTAINABLE FORAGING, WILDCRAFT AND RECIPES

DANIELLE GALLACHER

Contents

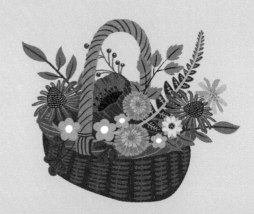

Introduction

The term 'wild' can carry a subconscious implication of the unknown or potentially risky. By labelling things as wild – swimming, camping or food – it may suggest an element of unpredictability or unfamiliarity, evoking a sense of caution or fear. In essence, though, wild food is simply food.

Our legacy of gathering from nature precedes the cultivation of crops, reminding us that its characterization is simply a reflection of our present perspective in this moment of humanity. Our ancestors relied on being able to identify and gather plants, fruits, nuts and fungi out of necessity for survival. This knowledge was passed down through generations, forming a fundamental aspect of daily lives. But that common knowledge is no longer so common, and it has become unusual to meet someone who can tell a dandelion from a hawksbit.

The shift away from this second nature in modern times can be attributed to agriculture and technology, altering our relationship with nature and leading to a decreased reliance on foraging for survival. Urbanization, supermarkets and the convenience of processed food were the nails in the coffin for our plant identification skills. There is a certain irony in how our pursuit of technological advancements has contributed to a disconnection from nature. The same technology that facilitated convenience and progress has, in many ways, led to a longing for the simplicity and tranquillity of natural surroundings. Recent booms in organic, renewable and 'eco-friendly' trends signal a return to a greener way of life.

I struggle to pin-point when I became a 'forager'. Playing with plants and flowers has always felt instinctual. As a young child I would make herbal potions and lotions, and perfumes from floral water, and in preadolescent years I was often labelled a 'tomboy' – a word I disliked as much then as I do now – spending my days climbing trees, building dens, seeking out poisonous plants and eating hedgerow berries with my brother, as instructed by our childhood bibles, *The Dangerous Book For Boys* and *The Boys' Book of Survival*. As a teenager I was fascinated by mushrooms, spending many hours studying and drawing them. Then, while I was at art college, the *Ray Mears Bushcraft* series aired. My housemate and I were so inspired that we spent a

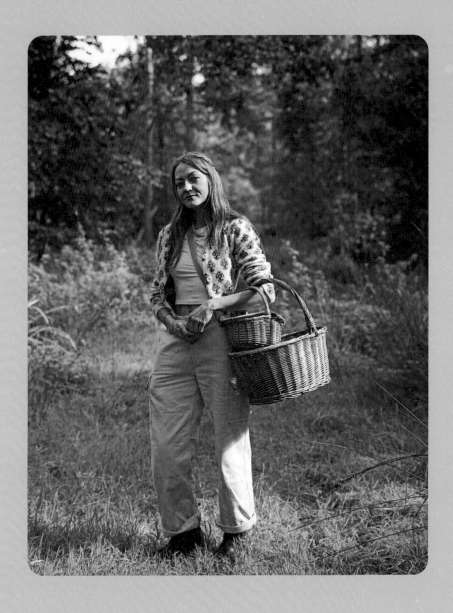

Cornish summer camping trip attempting to 'live off the fat of the land'– an unsuccessful feat that resulted in a meagre half a sandcastle bucket of limpets and two poorly bellies. Nonetheless, by this point, my love for wild food had very much taken root. I was hooked, and I hope you will be too.

About this book

I have been immersed in the world of wild plants and mushrooms for over two decades, teaching myself to forage through the simple joys of observation, sketching and growing a garden. After years of sharing my passion in-person through foraging workshops, herbal classes and nature connection retreats, I am now delighted to distil the experiences and knowledge I have gathered into this book for you.

We are, at our core, part of nature, and this guide is a gateway to not just observe it but actively participate in it, to taste it and to connect more deeply to it.

Starting with essential information on toxic species, useful tools and core knowledge, we then adopt a month-by-month approach to help you navigate the book; from year-round staples to my seasonal favourites, structured to

---

Gorse
Ulex spp.

A densely spiked evergreen shrub with cheerful yellow flowers known for their aromatic coconut scent, gorse can form impenetrable thickets, making them a valuable shelter for wildlife.

HARVEST TIME
All year round
FAMILY
Fabaceae
COMMON NAME
common gorse

Recognizable by its tough, sharp, furrowed thorns with bright yellow, pea-like flowers that grow in clusters on three-angled branches. The coconut scent gets more intense in the warmer months and can be used as a natural navigation method, as flowers on the south side of the bush will have a stronger coconut flavour than those growing on the north. The texture of the flowers is also reminiscent of coconut.

Traditionally, gorse has been used medicinally for its mild diuretic properties, to help treat digestive issues and as an antidote to melancholy. It can be used for weaving baskets and as a fuel for fires. The flowers can be used to make a fragrant tea, to help shift a glum mood.

Gorse is a perennial shrub with a few species, which extends the harvest time: common gorse (*Ulex europaeus*) flowers in the first six months of the year, with western gorse (*Ulex gallii*) and dwarf gorse (*Ulex minor*) flowering in the latter half of the year. All can be found in acidic environments, coastal areas, heathlands, meadows, open spaces and waste ground – don't forget your gloves!

LOOKALIKE: Scotch broom
(*Cytisus scoparius*)

Ground elder
Aegopodium podagraria

The arch nemesis of the gardener, ground elder is a hardy perennial that can have invasive tendencies, quickly carpeting damp, shady, nutrient-rich soils, lawns, woodlands and church grounds.

HARVEST TIME
Feb to May
FAMILY Apiaceae
COMMON NAMES
herb Gerard,
goutwort,
devil's guts

Ground elder can be identified by its ovate/elliptical pointed leaves on short stalks, which are three-lobed with a serrated margin. Leaves look somewhat similar to the elder tree (*Sambucus nigra*), the explanation for its common name. In summer, upright, hairless grooved stems bear flat umbels of small white flowers.

Young leaves and stems can be eaten raw, and buttered ground elder shoots was a common medieval peasant dish. Flowers can be used as a garnish and the dried root ground into baking flour. Once the plant has flowered, usually in early spring, the taste changes dramatically, as do the medicinal qualities, causing the plant to have laxative effects. Ground elder has also been useful in helping to treat inflammation, rheumatic pains and insect bites.

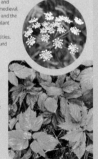

Spreading through rhizomes, ground elder can form dense ground cover. Be sure to collect only the youngest, freshest leaves for best flavour, as older leaves can leave you with a rather dreadful, lingering taste. The best time for harvesting is when the leaves are glossy, translucent and yet to unfurl – at this stage they have an inquisitive taste, somewhere between celery, carrot tops and aniseed.

LOOKALIKE:
☠ Dog's mercury (*Mercurialis perennis*)

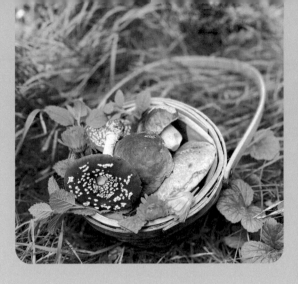

ensure you encounter plants and mushrooms at their zenith – whether flowering, fruiting or in abundance. Revisiting them at their various stages of life cycle unveils a deep understanding, fostering a relationship that goes beyond the conventional perception of plants solely as food.

This guide is suitable for greenhorn gatherers while offering nuanced insights for more experienced foragers. Key plants and mushrooms take centre-stage, each entry encapsulating not only their common and Latin names, identification features and harvest times but also an array of offerings and insights, inviting you to observe, learn and form bonds with your food and medicine. Scattered recipes and wildcrafting ideas extend an invitation to explore delicious and practical ways of befriending the flora and fungi around us.

In the opening chapter, we delve into a crucial aspect – cultivating an awareness of toxic species. As we learn about the beauty and utility of our green and fungal companions, recognizing potential hazards establishes a fundamental foundation. Although this initial step may feel challenging, it sparks a transformative shift in our perception, and instead of breeding intimidation, as one might expect, it instead unlocks a landscape where each plant and mushroom becomes a familiar face.

Toxic symbol ☠
Take caution with toxic lookalikes marked with this symbol ☠. All other lookalikes are edible, and I encourage you to do further research on those once you have finished with this book.

Getting started

Focus on the familiar

First things first! You should begin by identifying and learning about wild edible plants that are commonly found in your local area. Choose plants that resemble familiar cultivated vegetables or herbs, or wild greens you already know; for example, dandelion greens, nettles and some wild berries are often easily recognizable.

Begin with just a few types of wild foods that you're confident about identifying correctly, as this will help you build your confidence and knowledge over time. Learn the properties of each plant and the different ways you can connect with it, for example through food, medicine and wildcrafting. You might be surprised to learn that even the humble daisy has some potent medicinal properties.

Get educated

A good field guidebook (such as this!) is a must, as well as larger reference books to check further once you get home. Pay close attention to identifying features, growth patterns and any lookalike plants that might be toxic – we'll be delving into these a little later (see page 16).

Forage responsibly

Be careful not to disturb the surrounding flora and fauna when gathering wild foods – remember that the plants and fungi we forage are not only food to, but also homes to, thousands of species of wildlife.

Always forage in areas where it's safe and legal to do so. Avoid picking plants from polluted areas or places treated with pesticides, which, unfortunately, includes the borders of most agricultural land. Respect the environment by taking only what you need and leaving only your footprints.

Join groups or workshops

Local foraging groups, walks and workshops are a great way to learn from experienced foragers. No matter how many books you read, nothing compares to gaining hands-on experience.

Be seasonally aware

Different wild foods are available in different seasons. Familiarize yourself with the seasonal patterns of the wild plants growing around you. Growing a garden and cultivating wild plants is an awesome way to get to know their properties.

Add some wild ingredients

Start by incorporating wild foods into familiar recipes. For instance, you can add foraged greens to salads, blend wild berries into smoothies, or use edible flowers as garnishes. It's even possible to swap out your entire spice cupboard for foraged alternatives (see page 201).

Be open to experimenting with new flavours. Wild foods often have unique tastes, and exploring these can be a fun and exciting way to improve your cooking. It's also important to understand how localized certain flavours can be – no two blackberry bushes taste the same – so, if you don't like something on first try, be sure to test another plant, tree or bush in a different spot before you rule it out completely.

Some wild foods might benefit from cooking or processing to reduce bitterness or enhance flavour. Others, including most fungi, must be cooked before consumption. Research the best cooking methods for the plants or mushrooms you've foraged – there are plenty of ideas in this book – and remember that wild foods can taste vastly different plant to plant and tree to tree, depending on their growing conditions, local environment and many more factors we are yet to understand.

Record your experiences

Keep a foraging journal to document your experiences. Note where and when you found each plant, how you prepared it and your impressions of taste and texture. This is also helpful for recording those tastier bushes, or keeping an eye on a promising mushroom patch the following year.

Connect with nature

Foraging is not just about food: it's also a way to connect with nature and the seasons. Embrace the meditative aspect of being outdoors and engaging with the environment. The land has a lot to teach us – not just about the wonders of its landscape, but also about ourselves.

Safety first

It's crucial to be certain of a plant's identification before consuming it. Some edible plants have toxic lookalikes, so be 100 per cent sure you can distinguish between them. The golden rule is: if you can't name it, don't eat it.

Patience and continuous learning are key when it comes to foraging and incorporating wild foods into your diet. Over time, you'll develop a deeper understanding of your local ecosystems and the seasonal delights they have to offer.

Foraging kit

ESSENTIAL ITEMS

Field guide A reliable and comprehensive field guide, such as this one, is essential for identifying plants and mushrooms in the wild. As you will find on the following pages, there should be clear photographs, descriptions and information on the habitat and seasonality of the species included.

Basket or bag A sturdy basket or bag is a great way to carry your foraged finds. Look for a lightweight and durable option with enough space for your harvest. I find that waxed canvas bags are ideal for wild greens, and I prefer mesh (or paper) bags for foraging mushrooms so that the spores can continue to drop as I walk across the woodland.

Gloves Thick gardening gloves are advisable for protection against thorns and other hazards.

Knife A small pocket knife helps with cleaner cuts, avoiding infections to plants and trees.

First aid kit It's always a good idea to carry a basic first aid kit with bandages, antiseptic and other essentials, just in case. (See page 202 for making your own wild kit.)

Appropriate footwear A comfortable and sturdy pair of shoes or boots is essential for navigating uneven terrain – you'll often find those perfect mushrooms in the most out of reach places, so it's best to be prepared.

Weather-appropriate clothing Anyone planning to be outdoors for a great deal of time should dress appropriately for the weather, with layers that can be added or removed as needed. Be sure to also wear long trousers and sleeves to protect against scratches, bites and ticks.

USEFUL ITEMS

Hand trowel or digging tool A small hand trowel or digging tool can be useful for digging up roots, bulbs or other underground parts of plants. Keep in mind that you must have the landowner's permission to uproot plants.

Notebook and pen Keep a notebook and pen handy for taking notes on plant identification, locations and other details while out and about.

Magnifying glass and pocket mirror A magnifying glass can help with plant identification, particularly when examining small or intricate details. I also keep a pocket mirror on me to look underneath mushrooms without having to pick them.

GPS or map Walking in the woods for hours can get a little disorienting, so you may find it helpful to have a GPS or map to navigate through unfamiliar terrain, or even to keep track digitally of foraging locations.

Camera Document your foraging finds with a camera, particularly if you're unsure about identification and want to take a further look at reference books back at home. Be sure to take lots of reference photos at all angles and of each feature.

Binoculars A pair of binoculars can be useful for spotting distant plants or wildlife, and can be particularly helpful when foraging for berries or fruits in trees.

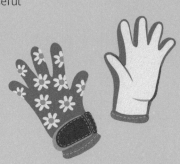

Identification tips:
What to look for

Habitat

Consider whether the plant grows in dry or wet environments, in forests or meadows, or in coastal or inland areas. Be sure to note the surrounding trees when searching for fungi.

Seasonality

The time of year in which a plant blooms or fruits can be a useful feature for identification. Consider whether the plant is a spring, summer, autumn or winter bloomer, and whether it fruits in early or late summer – though with climate change, this is starting to be less reliable.

Leaf shape

The shape of a plant's leaves can provide important clues to its identity. Leaves may be lanceolate (long and narrow), ovate (egg-shaped) or palmate (hand-shaped), among others.

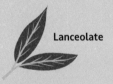 Lanceolate

Ovate

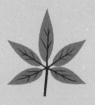

Palmate

Stem characteristics

Take note of the height, texture and colour of the stem. Is it grooved or smooth? Are there hairs or thorns? If so, are they soft or spiky?

Flower characteristics

Flowers can give us clues to species, family and even genus. Pay attention to size, shape, colour and scent. How are they arranged? How many petals are there? Which way do the sepals face?

Fruit characteristics

Fruit can be used to help identify plant species. Consider size, shape and colour, as well as any other distinguishing features, such as the presence of spines or hairs.

Growth habit

The way in which a plant grows can be a useful feature for identification. For example, some plants may grow upright, while others may trail along the ground or climb up other plants.

Geographic location

The location of a plant is also an important factor. Consider whether the plant is native to the area or whether it has been introduced from another region or country.

How to take a spore print:

A spore print is a useful part of the fungi identification process and can help us to corroborate our finds, however it should not be used as the only definitive guide as many fungi share similar-coloured spores. Once a mushroom has checked all other boxes for identification, you can then take a spore print for confirmation.

Cut the stem of a fresh mushroom close to the cap and lay the cap gill side down on a flat surface overnight. After a few hours the spores will start to drop, leaving a print that replicates the gill pattern. Scrape the spores together into a pile for a better idea on the overall colour. Some saprobic mushrooms can be cultivated at home by these spores.

Tip: Fresh specimens drop the most spores; however, if your mushroom is a little old, you can drip a droplet of water onto the cap to help the remaining spores release.

Toxic species

It is without doubt more important to learn what not to forage than it is to learn what to forage. This chapter lists the most dangerous plants and fungi that you could come across in the UK, a brief ID description, their edible lookalikes and some notes on their toxicity, too.

The words on the upcoming pages may seem daunting, but don't let them put you off. Foraging is perfectly safe (and thoroughly enjoyable!) when practised responsibly. There really aren't as many truly toxic species as one might expect, and a few are somewhat rare. Despite the infrequency of genuinely perilous acquaintances, it is nonetheless imperative to heed caution, and always advisable that inexperienced foragers search alongside a trusted and experienced guide, if possible.

Plant allergen test

Skin contact: Rub the plant part on a sensitive area of your skin, such as the inner wrist, inside elbow or outer lip. Wait for 15 minutes and observe any signs of skin irritation such as redness, itching, tingling or burning. If no adverse reactions occur, go on to the taste test.

Taste test: Chew a small amount (around a teaspoon) of the plant part for five minutes, spitting out saliva regularly. Wait for eight hours, monitoring for any delayed allergic reactions.

Eat a small amount: If there are no allergic reactions after the previous steps, progress to eating a larger quantity (one tablespoon) of the plant part. Wait for another eight hours, being vigilant for delayed symptoms. If all remains well, you can consider that specific part of the plant as safe for you.

Observation and caution: Throughout the testing process, be vigilant for any signs of allergic reaction, which may vary from person to person.

....

Caution
Symptoms of poisoning from plants and fungi include vomitting, stomach cramps, irregular heartbeat, burning to the mouth, lips or tongue and convulsions. The type and severity of symptoms will vary according to the type of plant or fungi, the amount swallowed and the size of the person.

....

Toxic fungi

Distinguishing between poisonous and edible mushrooms is impossible without accurate identification. There are many well-versed but entirely inaccurate and dangerous myths surrounding the toxicity of fungi but, truthfully, the only safe rule is to never consume anything unless absolutely certain of its identity. Listed here are the most toxic of fungi you're likely to come across, but remember that there are many more that could cause upset.

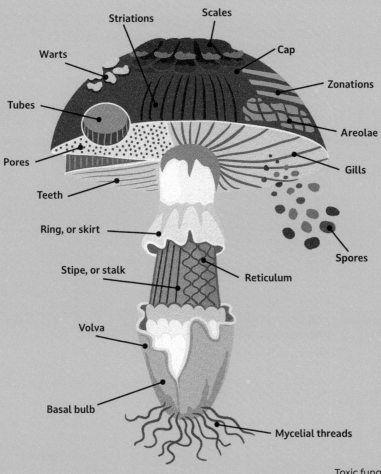

❶ DEATH CAP
Amanita phalloides

Appearance: Greenish-yellow in colour; indistinct snakeskin patterning on stipe; white gills are fairly broad, free and crowded. As an *Amanita*, the death cap grows from a sac-like volva and has a flowy 'skirt', or annulus, beneath the cap that is sometimes speckled with remnants of the universal veil, though this can be washed off easily by rain.
Size: Cap 5–15cm (2–6in) diameter; stipe 6–15cm (2¼–6in) tall.
Toxic effects: Severe liver damage, can be fatal.
Habitat: Deciduous woodland from August to November.
Spore print: White
Lookalike: False death cap (*Amanita citrina*)

❷ DESTROYING ANGEL
Amanita virosa

Appearance: Shares similarities with the death cap in both appearance and toxicity but is distinguished by its pure white colouring that can turn slightly off-white with age. Cap is usually smooth.
Size: Cap 5–10cm (2–4in) diameter; stipe 7–15cm (2¾–6in) tall.
Toxic effects: Ingestion of as little as half a small cap can result in severe organ failure and if left untreated there is a 50 per cent chance of death within a week.

Habitat: Uncommon, but found in woodland and glades from late July to October.
Spore print: White
Lookalikes: Edible agaricus, such as the horse mushroom (*Agaricus arvensis*) and field mushroom (*Agaricus campestris*) when in button stage.

❸ PANTHER CAP
Amanita pantherina

Appearance: Shiny ochre-brown cap coated in bright white fragments from its universal veil (membrane surrounding the baby mushroom). White gills are crowded and free. Beneath the cap hangs a prominent white skirt, smooth and without striations (unlike the striated skirt of the blusher mushroom). Shallow trough around the top of the volva.
Size: Cap 5–12cm (2–4¾in) diameter; stipe 5–12cm (2–4¾in) tall.
Toxic effects: Vivid hallucinations, confusion, delirium, convulsions and, in rare cases, death.
Habitat: Deciduous and coniferous woodland from June to November.
Spore print: White
Lookalike: Blusher mushroom (*Amanita rubescens*)

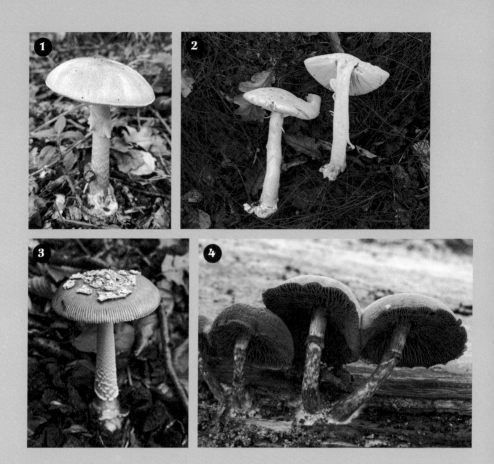

4 FUNERAL BELL
Galerina marginata

Appearance: Bell-shaped cap of young mushrooms later becomes convex or flat. Cap colour yellow-brown to dark brown with a sticky or slimy surface when wet. Crowded, tan-brown gills are attached to the fragile stipe, which features a brown ring, or annulus, although this is not always prominent on older mushrooms.

Size: Cap 2–8cm (¾–3in) diameter; stipe 2–8cm (¾–3in) tall.

Toxic effects: Deadly toxins, including amatoxins; ingesting even a small amount can lead to liver and kidney damage and, in some cases, death.

Habitat: Decaying wood, such as logs and stumps, June to November.

Spore print: Rusty brown

Lookalikes: Velvet shank (*Flammulina velutipes*), honey fungus (*Armillaria mellea*)

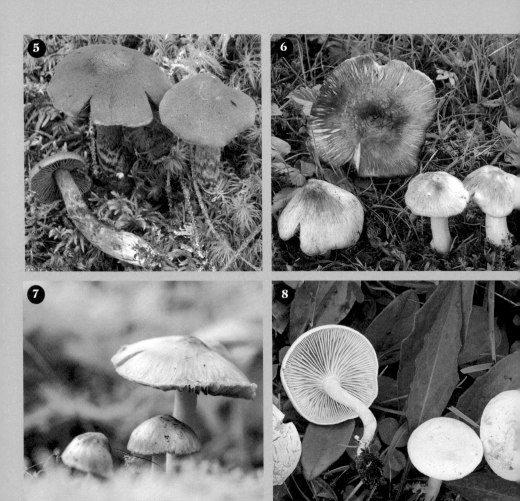

5 DEADLY WEBCAP
Cortinarius rubellus

Appearance: Rusty brown conical-shaped cap starting out with an in-rolled margin but flattening with age. When young, fine fibrils connect the stipe to the cap. Stipe is lighter in colour than the cap and is often curved or slightly bulbous, sometimes featuring a subtle snakeskin pattern. Fibrous flesh is pale cream and has a faint radish smell. Gills start pale yellow, turning rusty brown as the spore develops.

Size: Cap 2.5–8cm (1–3¼in) diameter; stipe 5.5–11cm (2¼–4¼in) tall.

Toxic effects: Orellanine is the poison responsible for the intense flu-like

symptoms that include headaches, vomiting, kidney and liver failure and, in some cases, death.
Habitat: Acidic environments – coniferous woodland, among bilberry bushes and heather plants, August to December.
Spore print: Reddish brown
Lookalike: Fool's webcap (*Cortinarius orellanus*)

❻ DEADLY FIBRECAP
Inosperma erubescens

Appearance: Conical creamy white cap that flattens and stains tan to reddish brown with age; covered with fine fibrils. Stipe is the same colour and also reddens with age. Crowded cream-coloured gills stain reddish brown where touched. The mushroom has a sweet smell.
Size: Cap 3–7cm (1–2¾in) diameter; stipe 7–10cm (2¾–4in) tall.
Toxic effects: Contains muscarine, which can cause excessive sweating, vomiting, diarrhoea and, in serious cases, a fatally slow heartbeat.
Habitat: Deciduous woodland, commonly with beech and oak, May to October.
Spore print: Brown
Lookalike: St George's mushroom (*Calocybe gambosa*)

❼ LILAC FIBRECAP
Inocybe geophylla var. *lilacina*

Appearance: Lilac cap is round, starting off conical then flattening but keeping the distinctive umbo

(raised area in the centre of mushroom cap) and silky fibres. Stipe is also lilac. Purple hue fades as the mushroom matures.
Size: Cap 1–4cm (¾–1½in) diameter; stipe 6cm (2¼in) tall.
Toxic effects: Contains muscarine, which can cause sweating, stomach pains and excessive salivation.
Habitat: Deciduous woodland, roadside verges.
Spore print: Brown
Lookalike: Amethyst deceiver (*Laccaria amethystina*)

❽ FOOL'S FUNNEL
Clitocybe rivulosa

Appearance: Buff white mushroom starting off convex and flattening with age, often funnel shaped with a wavy in-rolled margin. Adnate gills can be slightly decurrent, white but turning dull with age. Stipe is the same colour as the cap.
Size: Cap 1–7cm (¼–2¾in) diameter; stipe 2–4cm (¾–1½in) tall.
Toxic effects: Intense vomiting, diarrhoea, heavy breathing, blurred vision and, in severe cases, can be fatal.
Habitat: In fairy rings, June to December.
Spore print: White
Lookalikes: Snowy waxcap (*Cuphophyllus virgineus*), St George's mushroom (*Calocybe gambosa*), fairy ring champignon (*Marasmius oreades*)

❾ ANGEL WINGS
Pleurocybella porrigens

Appearance: Pure white funnel-shaped fungus with a smooth cap and lobed margin.
Size: Cap 2–12cm (¾–4¾in) diameter. Can appear to have no stipe but it is often just very short. White gills and thin, white flesh.
Toxic effects: Contains chemicals toxic to the brain and can cause permanent brain injury.
Habitat: Grows in clusters on decaying conifers/from moss-covered wood, July to December.
Spore print: White
Lookalike: Oyster mushroom (*Pleurotus ostreatus*)

❿ YELLOW STAINER
Agaricus xanthodermus

Appearance: Starts off a brilliant white, turning off-white. When in button stage, the free, very crowded off-white gills are protected by a partial veil that lacks the distinct cogwheel patterning of some of the edible *Agaricus* species. Gills later turn pink and then a grey-brown as the spores begin to drop. The stocky white stipe quickly turns a vibrant yellow, particularly at the base. Strong smell of ink or phenol.
Size: Cap 5–16cm (2–6¼in) diameter; stipe 5–12cm (2–4¾in) tall.
Toxic effects: Nausea, stomach cramps, sweating and vomiting.
Habitat: Parks, gardens and under hedgerows, either singularly or in small troops, May to November.
Spore print: Dark brown
Lookalikes: Horse mushroom (*Agaricus arvensis*), field mushroom (*Agaricus campestris*)

⓫ COMMON INKCAP
Coprinopsis atramentaria

Appearance: Bell-shaped cap in shades of brown, usually with a darker umbo, blackening and liquifying from the cap margin.
Size: Cap 3–10cm (1–4in) diameter; stipe 5–17cm (2–6¾in) tall.
Toxic effects: Temporary sickness and delirium if alcohol is consumed 24 to 48 hours either side of ingestion, as contains coprine, a mycotoxin that inhibits the breakdown of alcohol in the liver.
Habitat: Parks and woodlands, June to November, though sometimes earlier with a wet spring.
Spore print: Black
Lookalikes: Other inkcaps

⓬ MAGPIE INKCAP
Coprinopsis picacea

Appearance: Starts as a white egg-shaped mushroom, growing to reveal bell shape and charcoal-brown/bluey-black colouring. Fluffy white tufts from the veil decorate the cap and can be washed off with rain. Free gills are crowded and white before blackening. Within 48 hours the mushroom dissolves into an inky liquid in an auto-digestive process called deliquescence.

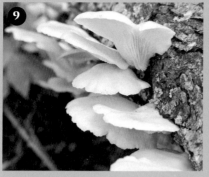
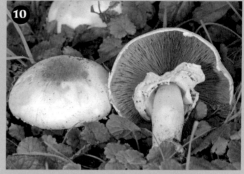
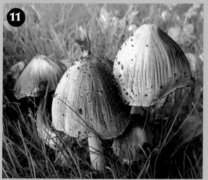
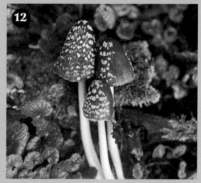
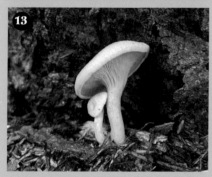

Size: Cap up to 8cm (3in) diameter; stipe 12–20cm (4¾–7¾in) tall.
Toxic effects: Nausea, vomiting and diarrhoea.
Habitat: Alkaline soil, grasslands and woodlands, August to December.
Spore print: Black

⑬ FALSE CHANTERELLE
Hygrophoropsis aurantiaca

Appearance: Vibrant orange, starting out convex but flattening into a funnel shape, often keeping an in-rolled margin and uniform shape. Inside flesh is the same colour as the cap and stem. Gills are also bright orange, and are deeply decurrent and forked.
Size: Cap 1–8cm (¼–3in) diameter; stipe 2–5cm (¾–2in) tall.
Toxic effects: Stomach pain, digestive upset, hallucinations.
Habitat: Coniferous woodland, July to November.
Spore print: White
Lookalikes: Chanterelles

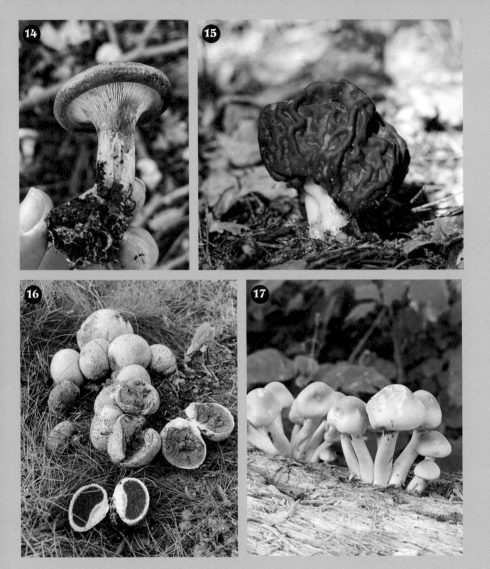

⑭ BROWN ROLL-RIM
Paxillus involutus

Appearance: Downy clay-coloured cap starts off convex, flattening with age, turning a deeper brown and developing a depression with central umbo. Cap margin is in-rolled; gills are a lighter shade of brown to the cap, darkening as the spores develop and staining brown where damaged. Stipe is fairly robust.

Size: Cap up to 15cm (6in) diameter; stipe 5–12cm (2–4¾in) tall.

Toxic effects: Immediate gastric

upset from improperly prepared mushrooms; cumulative effects from unknown toxin that causes haemolytic anaemia, a life-threatening autoimmune syndrome.
Habitat: Ectomycorrhizal fungi found in both deciduous and coniferous woodland, July to November.
Spore print: Orangey-brown

⑮ FALSE MOREL
Gyromitra spp.

Appearance: Resembling brains, with their irregularly lobed structure; usually a reddish or tan brown. The inside flesh is full of irregular chambers and hollows.
Size: Cap 5–12cm (2–4¾in) diameter; stipe 3–6cm (1–2¼in) tall.
Toxic effects: Contains gyrotoxins said to build up in the body, causing stomach pains, sweating, vomiting and even coma.
Habitat: Woodland, parks and gardens, March to August.
Spore print: Yellow to tan
Lookalikes: Many of the *Morchella* species

⑯ COMMON EARTHBALL
Scleroderma citrinum

Appearance: White balls attached by a mycelial thread in the ground. If you cut a young earthball, inside you will see a thick skin and an off-white inner flesh, which later turns a deep grey-purple, almost black, before the mushroom loses its tough, firm structure. When the spores finally mature, the loose skin explodes, enabling spores to puff out when disturbed.
Size: 3–10cm (1–4in) diameter, but can reach 15cm (6in).
Toxic effects: Abdominal pain, vomiting and diarrhoea.
Habitat: Woodland, parks, ditches and gravel tracks, in huge numbers June to December.
Spore print: Dark brown
Lookalikes: Puffballs

⑰ SULPHUR TUFT
Hypholoma fasciculare

Appearance: Sulphur yellow, convex, umbonate cap with crowded, adnate, olivaceous gills. Stipe is a similar colour to the cap. Stipe is often curved or irregular shaped as they grow in clusters.
Size: Cap 2–8cm (¾–3in) diameter; stipe 5–12cm (2–4¾in) tall.
Toxic effects: Rarely fatal but can cause temporary paralysis, distorted vision and sickness.
Habitat: Very common, growing on dead wood, fallen trunks and dying stumps in all frost-free months.
Spore print: Purple-brown
Lookalikes: Honey fungus (*Armillaria* spp.), velvet shank (*Flammulina velutipes*)

Toxic plants

While there are some seriously dangerous plants on this list, try not to fear them too much, because once we learn what species or parts of the plant we must not eat, the rest of the learning journey comes down to curiosity and experimentation.

❶ FOOL'S PARSLEY
Aethusa cynapium
Appearance: Pinnate, fern-like leaves on a grooved, hairless and hollow stem. Umbels of small white flowers with five petals bloom in summer developing furrowed, egg-shaped seed pods in autumn. Has an off-putting smell when crushed.
Size: No taller than 60cm (2ft).
Toxic effects: Abdominal pain, a burning sensation in the throat, vomiting, convulsions, possible respiratory failure and coma.
Habitat: Open spaces, waste ground, fields, gardens.
Lookalikes: Wild carrot (*Daucus carota*), cow parsley (*Anthriscus sylvestris*)

❷ LORDS-AND-LADIES
Arum maculatum
Appearance: Broad arrow-shaped leaves and large, unusual flowers featuring a hooded leaf-like bract surrounding a tall spadix (spike) that develops bright orange berries in late summer.
Size: Up to 45cm (18in).

Toxic effects: All parts contain calcium oxalate crystals, causing pain and irritation in the mouth when chewed, and swelling and gastrointestinal issues if ingested.
Habitat: Woodlands, hedgerows and gardens.
Lookalike: Wild garlic (*Allium ursinum*)

❸ COMMON FOXGLOVE
Digitalis purpurea
Appearance: Rosettes of soft, downy leaves, broadly spear shaped, and tall spikes of colourful tubular flowers, most often in shades of purple and pink but also in yellow and white.
Size: Reaching over 2m (6½ft) high.
Toxic effects: Contains cardiac glycosides leading to arrhythmia and potentially death.
Habitat: Woodlands, meadows and gardens.
Lookalike: Primrose (*Primula vulgaris*)

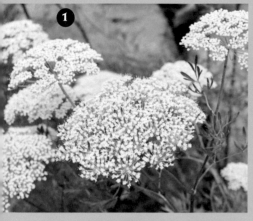

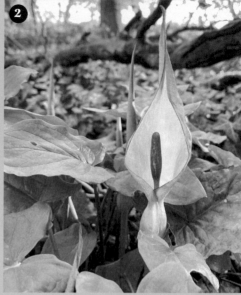

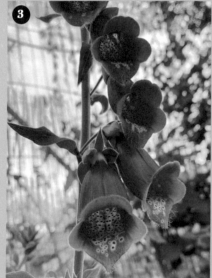

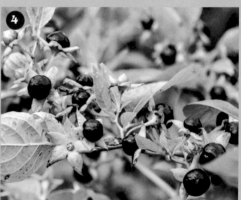

④ DEADLY NIGHTSHADE
Atropa belladonna

Appearance: Bushy shrub-like perennial with fragrant, brown or purple bell-shaped flowers and smooth, ovate leaves with prominent veins. In autumn, it produces shiny black berries surrounded by five large sepals that resemble a star.

Size: Up to 2m (6½ft).

Toxic effects: Contains tropane alkaloids causing rash, blurred vision, hallucinations, delirium and potentially fatal respiratory paralysis.

Habitat: Limestone and chalk woodlands, cultivated fields, waste ground.

Lookalikes: Potato plants

⑤ POISON HEMLOCK
Conium maculatum

Appearance: Branching biennial with smooth, green, hollow stems flecked with reddish-purple mottling, blotches or streaks. Bright green fern-like pinnate leaves with a serrated margin give off a musty aroma when crushed. Produces umbels of tiny white flowers with five petals.

Size: Upward of 2m (6½ft).

Toxic effects: Contains potent neurotoxins potentially leading to respiratory failure, coma and even death, with symptoms such as lack of coordination, salivation and trembling appearing in as little as 20 minutes.

Habitat: Sunny areas, meadows, disturbed areas, riverbanks.

Lookalikes: Wild carrot (*Daucus carota*), parsley (*Anthriscus sylvestris*)

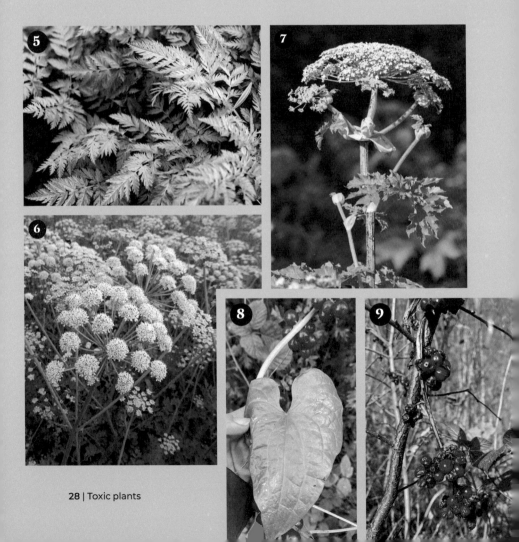

6 HEMLOCK WATER DROPWORT
Oenanthe crocata

Appearance: Pinnate, fern-like leaves on smooth, grooved and hollow stems. Compound umbels of small white flowers with five petals resemble pompoms and develop into clustered seed heads.

Size: Up to 1.5m (5ft).

Toxic effects: All parts are highly toxic, containing deadly neurotoxins triggering convulsions and respiratory failure.

Habitat: Wetlands, ditches and water margins.

Lookalikes: Wild celery (*Apium graveolens*), cow parsley (*Anthriscus sylvestris*)

7 GIANT HOGWEED
Heracleum mantegazzianum

Appearance: Gargantuan short-lived invasive perennial with a deep tap root, growing with huge, deeply lobed leaves forming jagged points, with green stems covered in bristles and flecked with reddish-purple streaks or blotches. Large umbels of white flowers with five petals develop into flat, oval seeds.

Size: Up to 5m (16½ft).

Toxic effects: Sap can cause severe burns, boils, blistering and skin irritation that can persist for years due to reactivation upon exposure to sunlight.

Habitat: Roadsides, riverbanks, disturbed areas.

Lookalike: Common hogweed (*Heracleum sphondylium*)

8 BLACK BRYONY
Dioscorea communis

Appearance: Twisting, climbing vine growing with large heart-shaped leaves and small greenish-yellow flowers with six petals that bloom in summer. Strings of glossy, bright red berries appear in autumn and can be seen into winter.

Size: Over 3m (10ft).

Toxic effects: Contains calcium oxalate crystals causing gastrointestinal upset if ingested and may also cause skin irritation upon contact.

Habitat: Hedgerows, field edges and woodlands.

Lookalike: White bryony (*Bryonia dioica*)

9 WHITE BRYONY
Bryonia dioica

Appearance: Climbing hedgerow vine with greenish five-petalled flowers in summer and orange-red berries in autumn, with slightly larger flowers and palmate leaves with five lobes.

Size: Over 3m (10ft).

Toxic effects: Contains bryonin causing nausea, vomiting and severe poisoning.

Habitat: Hedgerows, field edges and woodlands.

Lookalike: Black bryony (*Dioscorea communis*)

⑩ COMMON YEW
Taxus baccata

Appearance: Evergreen tree or shrub growing glossy needle-like leaves that lie flat and fleshy red cup-like fruits called arils that contain a large seed.
Size: Up to 20m (65ft).
Toxic effects: Contains toxic alkaloids that can cause heart failure; these are present in all parts of the tree except the fleshy red berries, which are in fact delicious, if not a little slimy. However, great care must be taken to remove the large seeds before eating as these contain high levels of poisonous taxine alkaloids, fatal in even small doses.
Habitat: Ancient woodlands, parks, church/abbey grounds.
Lookalikes: Other conifer species

⑪ HENBANE
Hyoscyamus niger

Appearance: Rough, hairy and sticky plant with pale yellow trumpet-shaped flowers with a pretty purple vein-like pattering and dark centres. Flowers bloom in midsummer atop single-stemmed plants. Broad and deeply lobed greyish-green leaves have a regimented appearance.
Size: Up to 1m (3ft).
Toxic effects: Contains tropane alkaloids, leading to hallucinations, delirium and potentially fatal respiratory paralysis.
Habitat: Waste or disturbed ground, along roadsides.

Lookalike: Deadly nightshade (*Atropa belladonna*)

⑫ SPURGE LAUREL
Daphne laureola

Appearance: Upright shrub with glossy, dark green alternate leaves and clusters of fragrant yellowish-green four-petalled tubular flowers that bloom in winter and develop into shiny, black egg-shaped berries in late summer.
Size: Up to 1.5m (5ft).
Toxic effects: All parts of the plant contain powerful toxins, the key compound being a strong irritant called daphnin causing nausea, vomiting and digestive irritation. Exposure can occur through skin contact with the sap causing blisters, rash and intense itching; the inhalation of sap droplets causes respiratory issues; ingestion causes abdominal pain, vomiting seizures, coma and possible death.
Habitat: Limestone woodland in both sunny and shaded areas.
Lookalikes: Other species of spurge, all of which emit a toxic sap

⑬ WOLFSBANE
Aconitum napellus

Appearance: A beautiful perennial herb with palmately lobed leaves and spiked racemes of strongly scented, hooded, indigo flowers arranged in whorls of three.
Size: Up to 1m (3ft).

Toxic effects: All parts, especially the roots, contain the powerful neurotoxins aconitine and aconine, which affect the nervous system, causing symptoms such as hallucinations, nausea, vomiting, convulsions, coma and death. Poisoning can occur by ingestion or absorption through nicks in the skin. One of the deadliest plants in the world, it can be fatal even in tiny amounts.

Habitat: Uncommon outside of gardens but can be found in woodlands, meadows and shaded banks.

Lookalikes: Common foxglove (*Digitalis purpurea*), mugwort (*Artemisia vulgaris*)

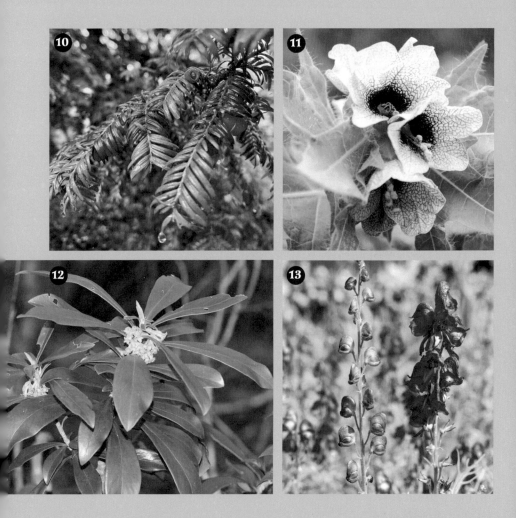

January

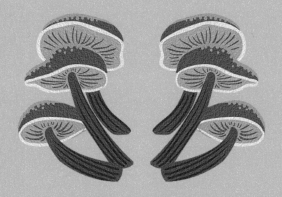

In the midst of brief daylight and seemingly perpetual nights, it can feel arduous to venture out into the frosty wilderness in search of wild food, and on first glance it would appear there is little substantial enough to garnish a plate, let alone fill the basket. But, take a closer look and you may start to notice the subtle signs of winter loosening her grip, or hear the soft whispers of those warmer days ahead.

Ground ivy, hedge garlic and winter cress can be spotted sheltering in pockets of woodlands and waste ground, and tree stumps are adorned with colourful turkey tail mushrooms.

At this time of year I tend to gravitate towards the forests and woodlands, seeking both refuge from the harsh winter elements and comfort from ancient trees. Although, there is often more wild food to be found in the fields at this time of year, and those who muster the bitter resolve of the January winds for long enough are sure to find it. If you've got a good eye you may just spot the young fresh leaves of overwintering plants such as chickweed and sorrel hidden among the overgrown tufts of grass. Beneath the soil lie plump roots of dandelion and burdock – brewing a batch of root beer is one of the most delightfully alchemic ways to spend a rainy winter's day.

Velvet shank

Flammulina velutipes

HARVEST TIME
Nov to Mar
FAMILY
Physalacriaceae
COMMON NAME
Velvet foot
SPORE PRINT
Cream

One of the best winter mushrooms, and hardy little things too, velvet shanks are able to withstand freezing temperatures, and even thrive when capped with snow! They're well worth the forage on a cold winter's day, not only for the flavour but also for the immune-system benefits they offer.

Velvet shanks have an orangey, caramel-coloured cap, which can range from shiny to mat depending on weather conditions. The velvety, ringless stipe is a pale orange colour on younger mushrooms, blackening from the base as they age in an ombré effect. The evenly spaced gills are cream coloured.

Boasting antioxidant, anti-tumour and anti-inflammatory properties, velvet shanks help to support and strengthen the immune system. They have a sweet, bready or biscuit-like flavour and are one of the few mushrooms that are safe to eat raw. A common way to cook them is to fry the caps in butter; the stems can be a little woody so are best used for stocks and soups. They keep well for a few days in the fridge, and can be preserved by drying or pickling.

A saprobic mushroom, it is found growing in clumps or tufts from dead, dying or diseased deciduous trees in late autumn to early spring, most notably elm but also on beech, oak, ash, sycamore and chestnut.

LOOKALIKES: ☠ Funeral bell (*Galerina marginata*),
☠ sulphur tuft (*Hypholoma fasciculare*)

Jelly ear
Auricularia auricula-judae

Do you ever get the feeling the trees are listening? Ear-shaped lobes of rubbery jelly give this fungus the appropriate common names of jelly ear and wood ear, and it is found throughout much of the year.

HARVEST TIME
All year-round
FAMILY
Auriculariaceae
COMMON NAME
Wood ear
SPORE PRINT
White

These easily recognizable auricular fruiting bodies jiggle either singularly or in clusters from the branches of the elder all year-round. Their translucent nature means the brown colour can seem variable, ranging from chestnut to russet or terracotta, depending on how the sunlight hits.

Jelly ears don't have much flavour of their own, but they soak up flavours well, so are useful in soups and stir fries, being a valued mushroom in Chinese cuisine for their immune-boosting properties. As drying is the most common form of preservation for these mushrooms, jelly ear can be harvested at any time, either when plump and fleshy or when dry and crispy. Rehydrate in a homemade rose-petal liquor or roll in dark chocolate for a foraged take on Turkish delight.

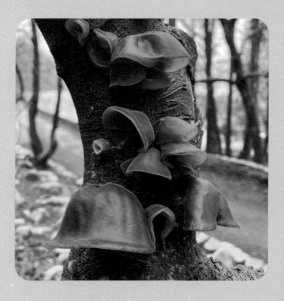

This is an abundant mushroom in the colder months, when fungi pickings are slim. Distinguish jelly ear from other more brittle cup fungi by the tree host (elder); their fuzzy outer surface; a smooth, shiny, veined inner surface; and their downward growth habit.

LOOKALIKES:
Peziza spp.,
leafy brain fungus
(*Tremella foliaceae*)

Wood avens

Geum urbanum

HARVEST TIME
Nov to Aug
FAMILY
Rosaceae
COMMON NAMES
Herb bennet,
colewort

With its recognizable upright branching stems, wood avens is a common perennial wildflower with a curious flavour profile – its roots are aromatic and spicy, so make a great alternative to cloves, cinnamon and nutmeg.

The branching stems bear small, five-petalled yellow flowers and three-lobed, greyish, toothed leaves. The round brown seed burrs are spiked with tiny hooks, the roots long and straggly.

The roots and rhizomes are high in eugenol (the main chemical constituent of clove oil), which has antibacterial, antifungal and antioxidant qualities, as well as being helpful in treating gastrointestinal disorders and skin complaints, promoting oral health and providing temporary pain relief. The leaves can be crushed and used as a topical insect repellent.

Dry the roots slowly to preserve the volatile oils, and use them to flavour both sweet and savoury dishes. For a chai tea, steep dried roots in milk alongside magnolia petals, common hogweed seeds and Alexanders seeds; you can also add the roots into your mulled wine recipe, or grind to a powder and use as a baking spice. The flowers can be used as a garnish, and while the leaves are also edible, they are downy, so are best lightly cooked.

LOOKALIKES:
**Wild strawberry
(*Fragaria vesca*),
barren strawberry
(*Potentilla sterilis*)**

Harvest roots in late autumn through to early spring, when the plant's energy is being sent towards its rootstock and before it puts out lots of new growth in April. Gather leaves when young and tender; flowers in summer. Find wood avens in damp, shady areas, scrub, hedgerows, roadside verges and gardens.

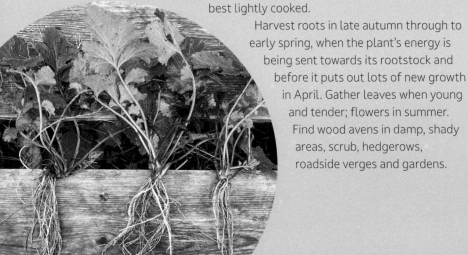

Hairy bittercress
Cardamine hirsuta

Widespread but often going unnoticed (unless growing in a garden, where it is unfortunately often labelled a weed) hairy bittercress is an underrated plant, neither hairy nor bitter, but rather pleasant with a peppery kick.

HARVEST TIME
All year-round
FAMILY
Brassicaceae
COMMON NAME
Flickweed

Look out for basal rosettes of pinnately compound leaves with a terminal lobed leaflet, small white flowers with four petals, and elongated spicy seed pods that explode when touched.

Rich in antioxidants and vitamin C, hairy bittercress has been used in herbal and folk medicine for its diuretic properties, helping to treat urinary tract complaints, and was also used as a treatment for poisoning and infections. As a member of the Brassicaceae family, it contains glucosinolates, which are known for their ability to remove carcinogens from the body.

Like most *Brassicas*, the seeds can be used for making mustard. Hairy bittercress offers a rocket-like hotness to salads, can be wilted like spinach or blitzed into pesto, while the flowers make for a graceful garnish.

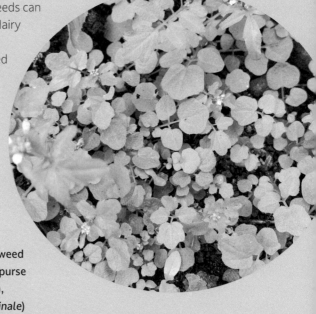

Hairy bittercress grows all year-round and loves damp, shady areas, well-trodden paths, waste ground and pavement cracks.

LOOKALIKES: **Common chickweed (*Stellaria media*), shepherd's purse (*Capsella bursa-pastoris*), watercress (*Nasturtium officinale*)**

Conifer trees

CONIFER ID TIPS

SIZE
Are the needles long or short?

SHAPE
Are the needles round, square or flat?

TEXTURE
Are the needles flexible or stiff?

ATTACHMENT
Are the leaves arranged singly, or in tufts or clusters?

Conifers provide valuable wild food, a medicine source and bushcraft uses all year-round: cordage can be made from the roots; insect repellents and antibacterial wound cleaners from the needles; and fire starters, glue, gum, plasters and incense from the resin.

Although they can all look similar at first, take a closer look and you'll soon be able to distinguish a spruce from a fir. Uses are often interchangeable between species, though you will find that flavours can vary dramatically.

Pine *Pinus*

FAMILY **Pinaceae**

Needles grow in fascicles (clusters) from a single origin point, are often soft and tend to grow to greater lengths than other conifers. Cluster size can help to narrow down species: two needles for red pines; three needles for yellow pines; five for white pines. Scots pine (*Pinus sylvestris*) is the only conifer with two twisted needles per fascicle.

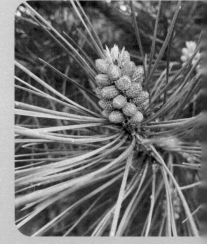

Pine needles contain antioxidants, including flavonoids and phenolic acids, and can be brewed into a tea to help relieve inflammation, chest congestion and circulatory dysfunction, and they have been shown to have memory-enhancing effects.

Caution
Be sure to steer clear of the deadly common yew, see page 30.

Long needles make beautiful weaved baskets.

The male cones begin to produce their pollen between March and May. Pine pollen is rich in macronutrients and bioactive compounds, can help boost testosterone and lessen fatigue. To harvest the pollen, pluck the young cones from the branches and place into a sealed jar, give it a vigorous shake, then sift through a fine mesh. Young cones are ready to harvest when they give out a puff of pollen when flicked.

The young cones make a delicious syrup called mugolio: layer green cones and brown sugar in a sterilized jar until full and leave to macerate in a warm, dry spot for three to four weeks, shaking and opening/closing the lid occasionally. Once the month is up, pour the contents into a pan and heat until the sugar is dissolved. Strain and decant into your container, and store in the fridge. Mature cones turn reddish-brown or black, becoming stiff and woody – excellent for tinder!

Larch *Larix*

FAMILY **Pinaceae**

The only deciduous conifer in Europe, larch trees turn a stunning golden hue in autumn. They have soft tufts or rosettes of needles all along the branches. The new bright green growth can be harvested and used for tea to lower cholesterol and boost the immune system. Larch also produces pink, edible 'larch roses': try dipping these in egg wash (or the juice from a tin of chickpeas) and rolling in sugar for crystallized cake decorations, or add them to a pan alongside sugar or honey for a zesty larch rose syrup.

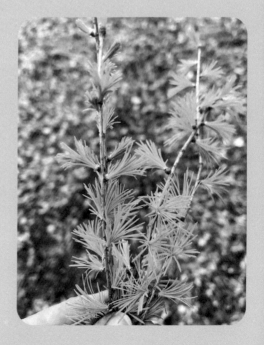

Spruce *Picea*

FAMILY **Pinaceae**

Needles are short, stiff and square, growing from a single origin point around the branch, and are attached to small, stalk-like woody projections, which remain behind when the needles are removed. Cones are smooth and flexible with thin scales, and tend to droop towards the ground.

Conifers produce a sticky resin packed full of essential oils and immune-stimulating properties. Try making a resin-infused oil by crushing 25g (¼ cup) of frozen resin in a pestle and mortar, adding to a jar with 100ml (3fl oz) of your chosen oil and placing in a pan filled with a few centimetres of water, simmering for at least 90 minutes to let the oil infuse. Be sure to keep an eye on the water level! Strain the oil into your container through a fine mesh while still hot. Use your oil for healing salves and lotions.

Fir *Abies*

FAMILY **Pinaceae**

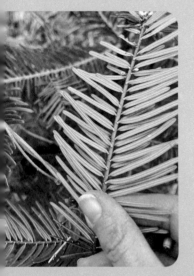

Firs are recognizable by their classic Christmas-tree shape. Flat needles grow from a single point of origin around the stem, similar to spruce, but are attached to the branch in a manner resembling a suction cup – when the needles are removed they do not leave behind a woody projection. Soft cones grow upwards like candlesticks and can be purple, green or blue, before changing to a golden brown.

Fir species are most likely to be confused with common yew; however, the underside of fir needles feature two silver parallel lines and have a citrus-like aroma when crushed, unlike the dull or matt undersides of yew needles. Add the antibacterial and antifungal fir needles to a spray bottle with vinegar for a forest-fresh all-purpose cleaning solution.

Juniper *Juniperus*

FAMILY **Cupressaceae**

An evergreen shrub with sharp needles grouped in threes around the ridged branches and which have a single pale band on the upper surface, with a greenish-grey underside. Juniper produces round, green berry-like cones, which turn fleshy and gain a deep blueish-purple colour, at which point they have a resinous sweet flavour.

Juniper is antibacterial, anti-inflammatory, antimicrobial and is prescribed as an herbal medicine for digestion problems and loss of appetite. Try fermenting berries to make the traditional Balkan bittersweet lemonade, *smreka*, by adding a couple of handfuls of juniper berries to a jar of filtered water with optional lemon slice/rind, sealing tightly and placing in a warm spot, then opening and stirring every few days for two to four weeks until aromatic and lightly carbonated.

Spruce resin firelights

1. Locate and collect your conifer resin, being mindful not to harm the tree while harvesting.

2. Gather dry sticks or chop pieces of fatwood into large matchsticks.

3. Melt the resin into a liquid over a low heat.

4. Dip your sticks into the resin – work quickly as it sets fast!

5. Once lit, the firelighters will burn for up to 10 minutes, giving you plenty of time to get a fire going.

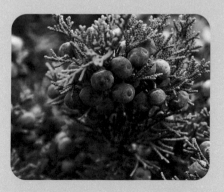

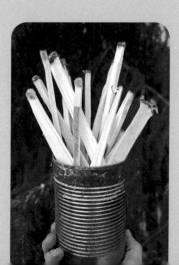

February

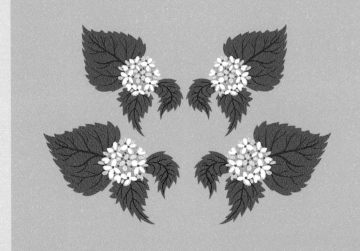

The first flowers are already showing: snowdrops, crocus and daffodils all casting an ethereal glow. Deep green blades of wild garlic start to push up from the dark forest floor, while rubbery jelly ear fungus and glossy caramel-coloured velvet shanks find their place on decaying trees.

Blackthorn gracefully takes the lead with blossom, covering the skeletal hedgerows with tiny white glittering flowers that shimmer under the late winter sun; and nettles, cleavers and primose are now growing large enough to spare a sprig or two. If you come across a magnolia tree, take a moment to run your fingers over the soft, fuzzy casings before the flowers burst open next month.

Squint just right and you'll catch a glimpse of the tiny female hazel flowers that will transform into clusters of delicious nuts come autumn, but it's from afar that the real changes of spring become apparent – there, on the horizon, the swelling tree buds wrap the distant woodlands in an enchanting purple haze, a sure sign that spring is on its way.

February is my favourite of months to harvest root crops: the heavy rain and frosts over winter really help to loosen up the soil, making a typically wet and dirty job a much less tedious task.

Three-cornered leek
Allium triquetrum

An incredibly easy plant for beginners to identify, especially when flowering, this grassy plant is unmistakable when crushed, giving off a strong garlicky scent.

White flowers have a green stripe down each of the six petals. It's not just the flowers that give this plant's identity away; it's also the cornered, grass-like leaves and flower stems, which, when cross-sectioned, appear triangular, hence the name.

The leaves, flowers, seeds and bulb of three-cornered leek are all edible, with the young, tender leaves or flower stems added to salads in place of spring onions or chives for their milder oniony flavour, or used to replace leeks in soup. The flowers buds are great pickled, with the opened flowers making for a pretty and tasty garnish. The seeds are also delicious, and can be used fresh and green or ground and stored as a spice when they are black and mature.

Found growing along walls, on woodland trails, in parks and gardens, on grass verges and banks, and, very often, in churchyards. Leaves appear in late autumn and early winter, flowering in early spring.

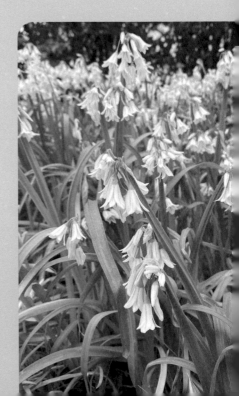

LOOKALIKE:
Few-flowered leek
(*Allium paradoxum*)

Caution
It is an offence to deliberately, or even accidentally, introduce this plant into the wild.
Be sure to use enclosed containers when harvesting so that flowers or roots do not accidentally escape when heading back home.

Alexanders

Smyrnium olusatrum

Alexanders used to be cultivated by monks in kitchen gardens, so lots of the 'wild' Alexanders we find will have escaped and reseeded from these historic grounds.

HARVEST TIME
Jan to Sept
FAMILY
Umbellifers
COMMON NAME
Horse parsley

Easily identifiable by the glossy, bright green trifoliate (in groups of three) leaves, the leaf base is always shrouded where it meets the main stem, which is thick, succulent and easily peeled, becoming hollow and grooved in more mature plants. The small umbel flowers are bright yellow/lime green and bloom from February to July.

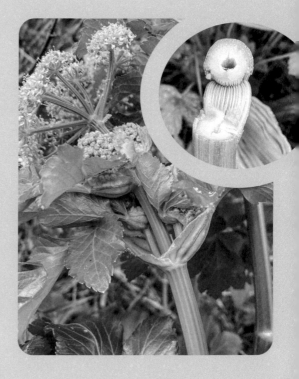

The entire plant is edible and was once a common ingredient, not dissimilar in taste to celery, though a little more floral. Leaves can be eaten raw in salads or steamed like spinach; stems can be peeled and boiled until tender or candied; flowers can be battered or used fresh in salads. In addition, unopened buds can be treated like sprouting broccoli and be pickled or fried. The seeds are slightly spiced and can be used to add an aromatic taste to stocks, soups and stews.

Alexanders are common in coastal areas, along sea walls and on land around old buildings.

LOOKALIKES: ☠ Hemlock water dropwort (*Oenanthe crocata*), wild celery (*Apium graveolens*), fool's watercress (*Apium nodiflorum*)

Fire cider

An age-old folk remedy to ward off winter illness, fire cider stimulates digestion and boosts metabolic heat. Sip a spoonful each morning to help wake and warm you up, and to ward off colds and flus, or use as a base for a salad dressing or even a (spicy!) shrub drink.

The standard base ingredients of a traditional fire cider include apple cider vinegar, garlic, onion, ginger, horseradish and hot peppers – however, this is my wild version! All ingredients are common plants that can be easily foraged from a wide range of habitats.

50g (2oz) three-cornered leek bulbs

25g (1oz) hedge garlic root

25g (1oz) horseradish root

25g (1oz) turkey tail mushroom

Handful of rosehips or hawthorn berries

Sprinkle of common hogweed seed

500ml (1 pint) apple cider vinegar

Honey

1. Wash, chop and place your foraged ingredients into a sterilized glass jar.

2. Top with apple cider vinegar so everything is fully submerged.

3. Shake well and store in a dark, cool place for four to six weeks, shaking every couple of days.

4. When you're ready to use, strain through a cheesecloth into a clean jar.

5. Add honey to your desired sweetness and stir until well mixed.

This recipe makes 500ml (1 pint) of fire cider, but you can adjust the ingredients and their amounts to the size of your jar, what's in season around you and/or which medicinal properties you feel would be beneficial to you over the winter months.

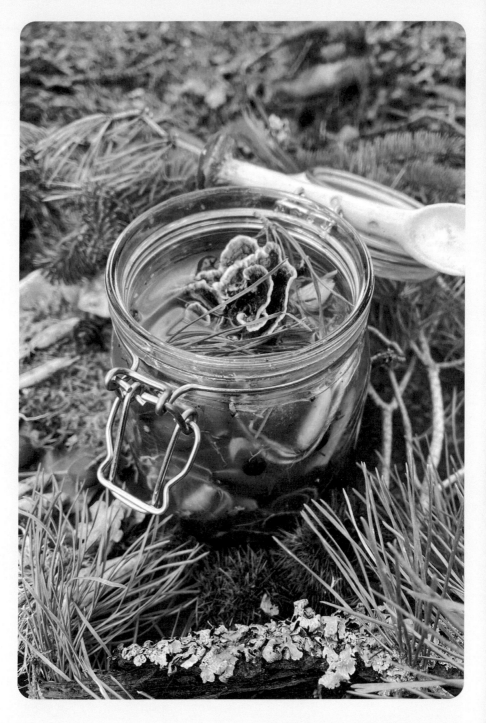

Dandelion
Taraxacum officinale

A common perennial plant with toothed leaves, the dandelion is known for its cheerful yellow flowers that turn into fluffy balls of silvery seed dispersing in the wind.

HARVEST TIME
All year-round
FAMILY
Asteraceae
COMMON NAMES
Lion's tooth,
blowball,
wet-the-bed

Dandelion forms basal rosettes of deeply lobed lanceolate leaves. Composite flowers with bright yellow petals radiate from a central disc and sit atop a long, hollow stem that exudes a milky sap. Flowers mature into spherical clusters of feathery parachutes.

The stem sap can be used to help treat acne, clear pores and remove warts. Traditionally used for its diuretic properties, dandelion can help to support liver health and digestion. Steep leaves and flowers in hot water for a tea that can help to

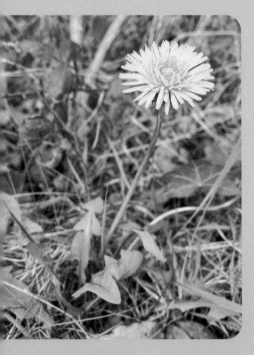

regulate blood pressure and sugar levels, balance cholesterol, detoxify the liver, support digestion and improve the immune system. Harvest young leaves for salads or, if you find them too bitter, they can be cooked as greens. The flowers can be used to make dandelion wine, and the long tap root roasted for a coffee substitute. Make dandelion syrup by boiling flowers with sugar and water, for use in cocktails, desserts or drizzled over pancakes.

Known for its resilience and adaptability, dandelion can be found all year-round in lawns, meadows, fields, gardens, parks and waste ground; it flowers from March to October.

LOOKALIKES: **Cat's ear (*Hypochaeris radicata*), hawkbit (*Leontodon* spp.)**

Hedge garlic
Alliaria petiolata

One of my favourite wild herbs to forage, hedge garlic is a lot milder than wild garlic but with a distinctly pleasant oniony-mustardy aftertaste.

Reaching 1m (3ft) once in flower, hedge garlic has kidney- to heart-shaped leaves and a blunt, irregularly serrated margin when young, becoming more triangular and nettle-like when older. They have prominent veins and emit an oniony garlic scent when crushed. Small white clusters of four-petalled flowers appear in the spring. After flowering, the plant produces elongated seed pods containing tiny black seeds.

The entire plant is edible and tops other *Brassicas* such as broccoli, kale and spinach in terms of nutrient density, containing vitamins A, C and E, omega 3 fatty acids, iron, manganese and calcium. Leaves can be eaten fresh or raw but are best harvested before the plant comes into flower in April or May. Add them to salads, sandwiches or to bulk out a pesto. Seeds can be ground up and used as a spice. Unopened flower stalks can be streamed or sautéed, or wait for the flowers to open and use as a garnish. The roots (best harvested between October and March) can be used fresh or dried, added to soups or finely chopped and used as a mild horseradish substitute.

Hedge garlic tolerates sun and deep shade, and is found in woods, fields, parks, alleyways and verges, most of the year.

HARVEST TIME
All year-round
FAMILY
Brassicaceae
COMMON NAME
Garlic mustard

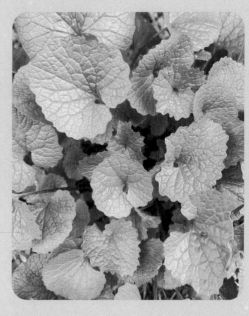

LOOKALIKES: **Nettles, other members of the Brassicaceae family**

March

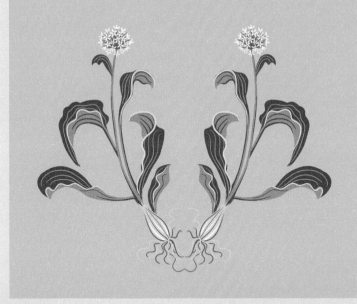

As the days lengthen and a gentle warmth graces the air, there's a palpable shift in the fields and forests. The mornings are now filled with a beautiful chorus of birdsong as the robin redbreast, blackbird, chiffchaff and blackcap guard their territories in anticipation of the upcoming breeding season, and small animals flit and scurry about as if energized by the promise of spring.

In many damp woodlands the dominant feature, and indeed scent, is that of the dense carpets of wild garlic. Shiny lobed leaves of ground elder can be seen poking through the crispy leaves, pale yellow primrose flowers speckle the forest floor and catkins hang elegantly overhead.

Trees and shrubs are now bursting their buds, with the bright green leaves of hawthorn being one of my favourites to snack on. Wild salad greens are aplenty, and for the next few months there's no need to buy lettuce or spinach. Look out for honesty, dead nettles, pink purslane and spring beauty all popping up – and, if you're lucky, maybe an early morel or two.

Birch

Betula spp.

HARVEST TIME
All year-round
FAMILY
Betulaceae

This common deciduous tree is known for its distinctive silvery-white striped bark, and green triangular-shaped leaves with serrated edges that turn yellow in autumn.

Harvest fresh, young leaves in spring for birch-leaf tea or vinegar, or infuse into oil for a topical salve to treat eczema and inflamed skin. Leaves can also be used to make a steam inhalation to help treat congestion.

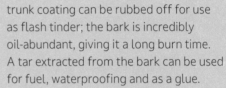

Birch trees are great for fire starting: the flammable papery trunk coating can be rubbed off for use as flash tinder; the bark is incredibly oil-abundant, giving it a long burn time. A tar extracted from the bark can be used for fuel, waterproofing and as a glue.

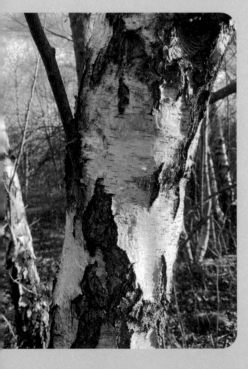

Around four weeks before the leaves appear in April, birch trees can be tapped for their nutrient-rich sap and enjoyed as a refreshing springtime tonic, reduced for a sweet and sticky birch syrup, or made into wine. Birch sap tastes just like water but with a slightly sweet flavour, which can be sweetened further by boiling and reducing by around a third, until the sap has a lovely amber colour, or keep on reducing to produce a thick, dark brown, sticky syrup. Making birch syrup requires time and energy – 50 litres/10 gallons of sap produces around half a litre/a pint of syrup – and is best done outside on an open fire. Store your birch water in the fridge for a few days; boil and hot-pour into mason jars for long-term storage; or freeze indefinitely. Syrup will keep for a few years in the fridge.

Japanese knotweed
Reynoutria japonica syn. *Fallopia japonica*

Japanese knotweed has a thuggish reputation, but its shoots and flowers are perfectly edible, sharing rhubarb's sourness, without the sweetness. Its reddish-purple shoots – reminiscent of asparagus spears and appearing in February – make it, thankfully, easy to identify.

The shoots unfurl to reveal thick, speckled bamboo-like canes that grow up to 3.5m (11½ft) tall with broad, shield-shaped, alternate leaves on zigzagged stems. Showy elongated clusters of creamy white flowers appear in late summer. The plant turns dry and bamboo-like, with noticeable hollow stems, in autumn that can persist throughout winter, with spring growth appearing through the old crown.

The shoots can be eaten raw or cooked in a similar fashion to rhubarb. Preserve by drying, freezing, turning into a syrup, or pickling in a water, salt and vinegar brine. Flowers can be used to make cordial or as a garnish.

Japanese knotweed is often found along riverbanks, roadsides and disturbed areas.

HARVEST TIME
Feb to Aug
FAMILY
Polygonaceae
COMMON NAMES
Fleeceflower, elephant ears, donkey rhubarb, Mexican bamboo

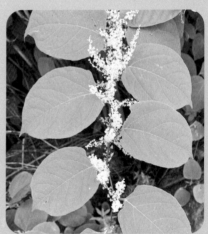

Invasive species
Not only can Japanese knotweed grow at a rate of 10cm (4in) a day, forming dense thickets, but it is also incredibly difficult to eradicate due to its deep pervading rhizomes. Labelled as an invasive species, it is important to take care when harvesting so as to not cause any spread of the plant.

LOOKALIKES: Himalayan knotweed (*Polygonum polystachyum*), giant knotweed (*Fallopia sachalinensis*)

Japanese knotweed & dog rose compote

I find no greater joy than cooking with invasive plants, and being a huge fan of rhubarb, the similar sourness of Japanese knotweed means it's a plant I find myself cooking with each and every year.

For this simple, sweet and sour-tasting compote, first you need to make a rose water, also known as a hydrosol, then the compote itself. Once made, safely stash your rose water in a bottle for use in cooking or cosmetics – it makes a soothing face toner. The compote is delicious served over pancakes, yoghurt or ice cream, as a cake filling, or stirred into custard.

Rose water:
A few handfuls of fragrant, fresh rose petals
Boiling water
Ice cubes

To make the rose water:

1. Place the rose petals in a large pot.

2. Create a makeshift still by nestling a small bowl among the petals.

3. Pour boiling water over the petals, being careful to avoid the bowl.

4. Seal the pot with an inverted lid, its handle facing downward.

5. Place ice cubes onto the lid and simmer for half an hour. Mop up melting ice with a dry towel, swapping for fresh ice as needed. (The ice is cooling the steam, causing condensation to form on the lid's underside; this condensed water then drips down and gathers into the empty bowl.)

6. Turn off the heat and carefully remove the bowl. This liquid treasure is your rose hydrosol.

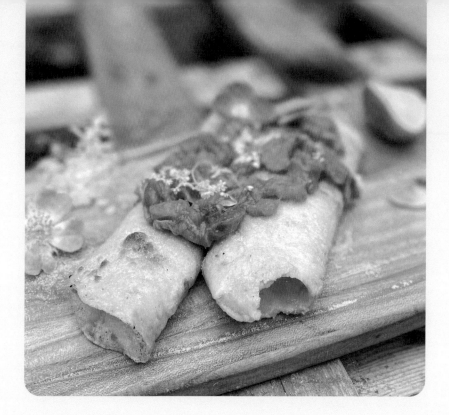

Compote:
500g (1lb) of young,
    fleshy Japanese
    knotweed shoots
300g (10oz) sugar
1 tsp rose water

To make the compote:

1. Rinse and chop the Japanese knotweed shoots into 2.5cm-long (inch-long) chunks.

2. Place into a pan with the sugar and heat until the sugar has dissolved, the knotweed has broken down and the mixture has thickened.

3. Remove from the heat and mix in the rose water.

Rock samphire
Crithmum maritimum

HARVEST TIME
Mar to Aug
FAMILY
Apiaceae
COMMON NAME
Sea fennel

A succulent maritime plant with fleshy stems and a salty carrot-like flavour, rock samphire is a tasty plant that will have you scrambling up the sides of cliffs to harvest – take care!

Rock samphire is identified by its branching stems with alternately arranged, fleshy, blue-green leaves and umbrella-like clusters of tiny yellow-green flowers that bloom in late spring to early summer.

A natural source of dietary fibre, rock samphire aids in digestion and helps to relieve bloating. Rock samphire is rich in unsaturated and saturated fatty acids and phytosterols, helping to moisturize the skin and reduce fine lines and wrinkles. The leaves, seeds and root were traditionally boiled in wine and used to treat urinary tract complaints.

With a pungent flavour similar to marsh samphire but with extra notes of carrot tops and lemon, leaves are best harvested in spring or summer before the plant gets too tough. Use to flavour foods in place of salt, eat fresh in salads (sparingly!), pickle for a crisp, tangy side dish or blitz up with butter for a salty, herby sauce. Preserve by pickling or lacto-fermentation, or infuse in olive oil for a flavourful dressing or dip to use in cooking or as a base for marinades.

Rock samphire thrives in coastal areas: on beaches, cliff tops and rocky shores.

LOOKALIKE: **Sea kale (*Crambe maritima*)**

Cow parsley
Anthriscus sylvestris

A delicate, lacy plant with fern-like leaves and sprays of frothy white flowers on tall stems, cow parsley is a common sight in meadows and along verges and hedgerows during late spring and early summer.

The grooved, hollow stems are green and often tinged a purple-red colour. They have short, fine hairs that can be hard to see but which give the stems a coarse, textured feel, unlike the smooth, blotchy stems of its toxic lookalike, poison hemlock. Crushing the leaves of cow parsley will reveal a subtle parsley-like aroma. It blooms in spring, with clusters of small five-petalled white flowers that grow in large, flat umbels.

High in vitamin C and antioxidants, cow parsley is often used for digestive complaints, to help alleviate headaches and for boosting the immune system. Its leaves can be applied topically as an insect repellent. The flowering buds are arguably one of the best parts of the plant, with a taste similar to parsley. Preserve the delicate flavour by pickling them in a vinegar brine. The crunchy celery-like stems can be eaten fresh or diced and added to soups, stocks and stews. The dainty flowers can be used as a garnish, and the seeds, too, are edible, with a carroty, parsley-type flavour – they are great as salad toppers or added into ferments.

Rosettes of pinnate leaves start pushing through in late winter to early spring, with the young flowering buds emerging around March and April.

LOOKALIKES: ☠ Poison hemlock (*Conium maculatum*), ☠ fool's parsley (*Aethusa cynapium*), ☠ hemlock water dropwort (*Oenanthe crocata*), wild carrot (*Daucus carota*)

HARVEST TIME
Feb to Apr
FAMILY **Apiaceae**
COMMON NAMES
Wild chervil, mother die

Caution
Be cautious when harvesting, as lookalikes include toxic species (see below).

Wild garlic

Allium ursinum

Wild garlic carpets the floor of ancient woodlands in spring and fills the air with an intoxicating oniony scent, you just need to follow your nose for this tasty wild green!

A pungent, bulbous perennial known for its long, broad, pointed leaves with a smooth, untoothed margin, the young leaves emerge in February and clusters of star-shaped white flowers with six petals appear later in spring, growing on the end of tall, thin stems. The entire plant has a strong onion-garlic scent.

Wild garlic boasts all the same health benefits as its relative cultivated garlic, regulating blood pressure and lowering cholesterol, reducing risk of heart attacks and strokes. It has antibiotic, antiviral and antibacterial properties, and contains vitamins A and C, alongside calcium, iron, phosphorus and sodium.

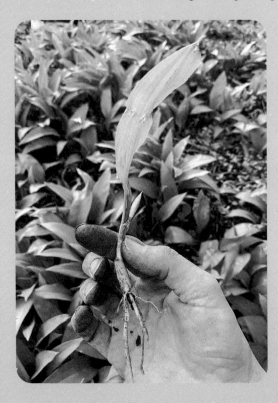

Harvest leaves before flowering for a more intense flavour; older leaves are best added to soups, stews, sauces and pesto. Preserve leaves in oil or vinegar, or blitz into butter and pesto. The flower buds have a stronger flavour than the rest of the plant and are great lacto-fermented or pickled in apple cider vinegar (see page 60). Stems can be chopped and used similarly to chives, while the flowers make a delicious garnish. Crunchy, green seed heads are the final act to look forward to in early summer – these can be pickled like capers and are

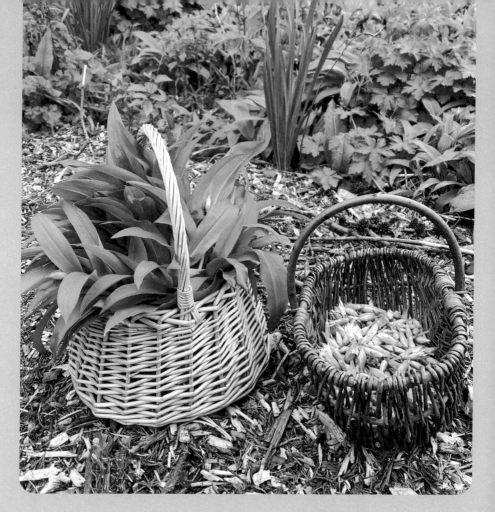

also perfect for sprinkling on top of any savoury dish. Bulbs can be used as a mild garlic substitute, but with so much flavour in the rest of the plant, you might have no desire to dig them up!

Common in damp, shady meadows, along streams and riverbanks, patches can stretch incredibly far throughout the woodland. However, it's important to not get carried away in the face of this abundance: be sure to pick only what you will use, as not only are wild garlic flowers an important early food source for bees, but badgers and wild boar also love to dine on the bulbs.

LOOKALIKES: ☠ Lily of the valley (*Convallaria majalis*),
☠ lords-and-ladies (*Arum maculatum*)

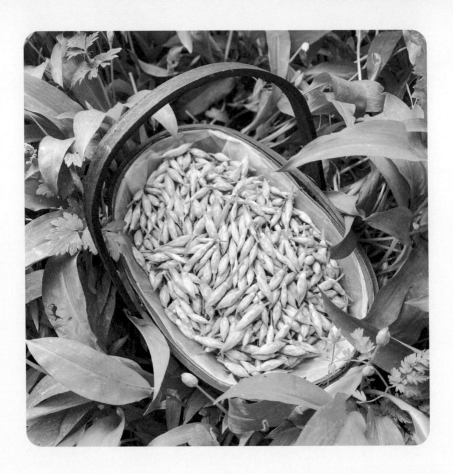

Pickled wild garlic buds

This is my favourite late winter/early spring recipe, and one of the easiest too. Wild garlic flower buds pack a punch, and one of the best ways to preserve their flavour for year-round gobbling is by pickling. I also like to mix up the flavours of my jars and add things such as sorrel leaves, chopped common hogweed stem, a few flowered leek bulbils, whole chillies, dandelion buds, and so on. It takes minutes to make and lasts all year.

Wild garlic buds
  (to fill jar)
Pickling vinegar
  (white wine or apple
  cider; to fill jar)
Brown sugar (to taste)
Salt and spices (to taste)

1. Sterilize a jam jar in the oven on low for 10 minutes. Leave to cool.

2. Tightly fill the jar to the top with garlic buds.

3. Heat the vinegar, sugar, a pinch of salt and the spices until the sugar dissolves. (I add things such as peppercorns, nigella seeds, mustard seeds, common hogweed seeds, chilli flakes or bay leaves, but add what you like.)

4. Simmer for a couple of minutes, then pour the vinegar mix over the top of the jarred buds until it reaches to just under the rim.

5. Leave to settle for a few minutes, then slowly stir to release any air bubbles.

6. Top with more vinegar mix to fill the jar, then seal with a lid and leave to get tasty for a month or two before opening.

Wild garlic butter

I've made a batch of this each March for most of my adult life – it goes in/on everything. The recipe could not be simpler.

A few handfuls of wild
  garlic leaves
500g (1lb) butter
Sprinkle of sea salt

1. Add the wild garlic leaves to a food processor along with the butter and a sprinkle of sea salt.

2. Blitz, roll up in parchment paper and leave to set in the fridge.

For the pickled buds, I love to mix up the flavours each year and usually add whatever I have at the time: a leftover slice of citrus peel; a few mustard seeds; some common hogweed seeds, which have flavours of citrus, cloves and cardamom.

Ground-ivy
Glechoma hederacea

Ground-ivy is a low-growing, creeping plant with a strong herby scent when crushed and leaves that give a powerful flavour.

HARVEST TIME
Mar to Nov
FAMILY
Lamiaceae
COMMON NAMES
Gill-over-the-ground, creeping Charlie, alehoof, tunhoof, catsfoot, field balm, run-away-robin

The stems of ground-ivy are square-shaped; the leaves dark green, kidney-shaped and scalloped. During spring, tiny, light purple flowers appear.

Ground-ivy can be used as a fresh poultice to help treat insect bites and nettle stings, and it is high in vitamin C and iron. It can be made into a healing tea to help relieve chest complaints and reduce inflammation. The flowers are also edible and ideal as a garnish. Add ground-ivy to salads as a bitter green to help aid digestion, or use it fresh for a strong-tasting herb to flavour or marinate foods; the flavour is less intense when dried.

Find ground-ivy in fields, meadows, woodlands, hedgerows and damp ground all through the year, although the leaves are best harvested spring through autumn.

LOOKALIKES:
Purple dead nettle (*Lamium purpureum*), henbit dead nettle (*Lamium amplexicaule*)

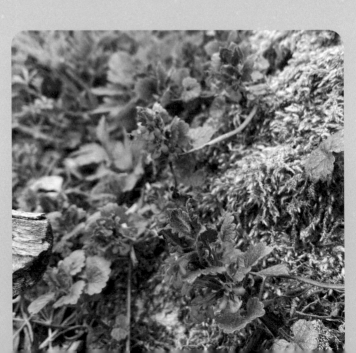

Magnolia

Magnolia spp.

The glorious magnolia is said to have been on Earth for 95 million years. With large, ostentatious blooms, the petals of this popular ornamental tree have an extraordinary spiced ginger flavour.

HARVEST TIME
Feb to June
FAMILY
Magnoliaceae

The flowers of the magnolia are often in goblet, bowl or star shape, some growing up to 30cm (12in) across, depending on the variety. Two of the most common species include the saucer (*Magnolia* x *soulangeana*), with tulip-shaped pink-blushed flowers and large, broad leaves; and the star (*Magnolia stellata*), with 12 or more white petals and smaller, narrower leaves.

Magnolia is an antioxidant and anti-inflammatory, and can also help to reduce anxiety. Flower buds and petals have a spiced ginger-like flavour and can be eaten fresh, infused into a syrup, added to spring flower rice rolls or dried for tea blends. Pickled magnolia petals make an awesome side to sushi as a replacement for sliced ginger: bring a mild vinegar, some sugar and salt to a boil, simmer until the sugar has dissolved, add a handful of petals into a sterilized jar and top with the cooled vinegar solution. Seal with a lid, leave to get tasty for at least a week and keep in the fridge for up to a year. Magnolia 'pineapples' (the spiral-arranged stamens) share the gingery flavour and make interesting cake toppers.

Though not all species of magnolia are listed as edible, there are no known toxic species. Not a wild or naturalized plant, magnolia is a popular ornamental tree in gardens and parks; if seen outside of a cultivated landscape, it will be an escapee.

Sweet woodruff
Galium odoratum

This low-growing, mat-forming perennial herb has whorled leaves and clusters of fragrant white flowers that seem to twinkle amid the shaded forest floor.

HARVEST TIME
Mar to Nov
FAMILY
Rubiaceae
COMMON NAMES
Sweet-scented
bedstraw

Deep green, elliptical leaves in whorls of six to nine grow up square stems with tiny, tubular, star-like white flowers with four petals on terminal clusters, blooming in June and July. Flowers develop into little balls of hooked bristles.

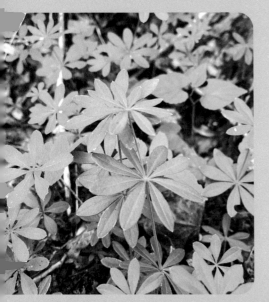

Sweet woodruff is antiseptic and can be used as a wound wash. You can also infuse it into dairy products or add it to herbal teas to help treat heart, lung, liver, stomach, gallbladder and urinary complaints. The subtle scent is due to the presence of coumarin, which not only lends its own sweet notes of spiced vanilla and fresh hay, but also has the ability to remove other odours from the air, making it great for potpourri or to hang in sprigs from your rear-view mirror; when dried the vanilla scent of sweet woodruff intensifies and can retain its aroma for years. It is often used to flavour alcohol, the most popular being May wine, which is drunk during spring solstice celebrations. The leaves and stems can be used to made a grey-green dye, while the rhizomes produce a red dye.

Found in shaded woodlands and beneath hedgerows from March through to the end of autumn, dying back in winter.

LOOKALIKES: **Other *Galium* species**

Shepherd's purse
Capsella bursa-pastoris

A common annual weed recognizable by its heart-shaped pods and orange seeds resembling coins in a purse, the whole plant is edible, with a peppery taste similar to rocket or mustard.

HARVEST TIME
Mar to Oct
FAMILY
Brassicaceae

With a basal rosette of deeply lobed leaves, though shape is variable, terminal raceme clusters of tiny, white, four-petalled cruciform flowers form in an opposite arrangement on smooth, thin, wiry stems. Upper leaves are sparse and lanceolate, with an untoothed or sparsely serrated margin. Flowers develop into heart- or arrow-shaped seed pods that, when dry, open up to expose the orange, elongated, oval seeds.

A well-known anticoagulant, it helps to reduce clots, heavy menstrual bleeding and haemorrhages. As part of the Brassicaceae family, shepherd's purse, especially the seeds, contains mustard oil glycosides, which are packed full of free radicals, anti-tumour agents and antioxidants, helping with viral infections, chronic inflammation, kidney stones and immune system support.

The immature green seed pods are arguably the best part to eat, with a spiced nutty flavour and slight crunch to them – they are fun sprinkled onto salads as people are usually amazed to discover that they can be gathered nearby. If you wait for the pods to turn brown and harvest the small seeds, they can be ground into flour.

Resilient and adaptable, you will find shepherd's purse in all manner of environments from fields, meadows and gardens, to disturbed areas such as car parks and pavement cracks. It blooms in early spring but can be found flowering throughout much of its growing season.

LOOKALIKE: **Shepherd's cress (*Teesdalia nudicaulis*)**

Lungwort

Pulmonaria officinalis

HARVEST TIME
Mar to Nov
FAMILY
Boraginaceae

This perennial with pretty pink and purple flowers, and a clumping growth habit, is noteworthy for its distinct silver or white foliage spots, thought to resemble diseased lungs and thereby cementing its use as a treatment for respiratory conditions.

Leaves are arranged in a basal rosette with an ovate to lanceolate shape, pointed tip, prominent veins running parallel to the midrib and a smooth leaf margin. Hairy stems give rise to clusters of tubular flowers, forming a nodding appearance as part of a cyme. Its flowers start life in pinkish or purplish hues, transitioning to blue or violet as they mature.

The doctrine of signatures is a concept in herbal medicine suggesting that if a plant resembles a specific body part, it can treat ailments related to that part. With the spotted leaves resembling diseased lungs, lungwort is used as an expectorant, helping to clear the airways and repel mucus from the lungs, and it has long been prescribed for asthma, bronchitis, catarrh and chronic cough. Leaves are high in mucilage, making them excellent as topical relief to burns, bites and sores.

The mucilage content means the leaves can turn mushy when over-cooked, so they are best lightly steamed, or shredded raw and added to salads. The pink and purple flowers make a lovely two-toned garnish for cakes and desserts.

Harvest leaves for food from when they first appear in early spring, typically March, or through to late autumn (typically November) for medicine. In sheltered spots in shady woodland areas you can find lungwort growing all year-round.

LOOKALIKES:
Other *Pulmonaria* species, borage (*Borago officinalis*)

Common comfrey
Symphytum officinale

Not only is comfrey one of the best plants for healing cuts and bruises fast, it is also a tasty food, a powerful fertilizer and a pollinator-friendly companion plant.

HARVEST TIME
Mar to Nov
FAMILY
Boraginaceae

This bushy perennial herb reaches nearly 2m (6ft) in height, with large, hairy, broadly lance-shaped leaves and drooping clusters of bell-shaped white, pink or purple flowers. Common comfrey can be differentiated by its strongly decurrent leaves that feature 'wings' that extend past the leaf below.

With a high content of allantoin, which promotes cell proliferation, a poultice made from crushed leaves helps ease wounds, bruises and sprains. It should only be used on cleaned open cuts, otherwise the cut can heal too quickly, trapping dirt and bacteria inside. Comfrey is a great source of vitamins A and B2, and K and K2, known for their blood-coagulant and bone-repairing properties. It also contains dietary fibre, manganese and rosmarinic acid, shown to have anti-inflammatory, antibacterial, antiviral and anti-tumour effects.

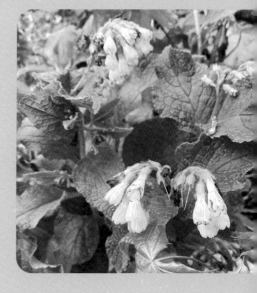

With a similar flavour to borage, think cucumber with a hint of watermelon. The leaves are rough-textured but can be eaten in salads when young. Steam stems as asparagus, and add flowers to salads and cakes. The large roots can be dried and ground as a coffee substitute.

Harvest leaves in spring before flowering; roots in autumn after flowering. Comfrey thrives in moist, fertile soil near rivers or streams and in woodlands, allotments and gardens.

LOOKALIKE: ☠ **Common foxglove (*Digitalis purpurea*)**

Comfrey & nettle bruise balm

You can use comfrey direct on the skin after a knock, fall, bruise or sprain, mashed up with a bit of water or whatever carrier oil you have to hand. However, making it into a salve is a much more practical (and less messy) application.

Nettles amp up the power of this healing balm, choose from white or red dead nettles, or even stinging nettles – all have healing properties that will soothe and enrich the skin. To make this balm, you need to have steeped dried comfrey and nettle leaves in your choice of oil. I've used hemp seed oil for a minimum of six weeks and strained the mixture. You can make the balm with just the oil and wax, or add a couple of extras such as shea butter and essential oils to tailor it to a specific application. Add vitamin E oil for extra nourishment and to act as a preservative, so your balm will last longer.

300ml (10fl. oz) comfrey
  and nettle oil
40g (1½oz) soya wax or
  30g (1oz) beeswax
Optional:
30g (1oz) shea butter
  (or coconut oil)
20 drops essential oils
1 tsp vitamin E oil

1. Melt the wax and comfrey oil together in a double boiler. Allow to cool.

2. Add essential oils and vitamin E.

3. Pour into your jar, tin or mould, and leave to set.

....

Note
The quantities of the ingredients you use can depend on what you have to hand and the preferred texture of the balm. The ones given here will make a soft balm that melts easily into the skin.

....

Comfrey is so good at healing that it's important to note that this balm should not be used on any wounds deeper than a scratch. It can cause cells to replenish so fast that bacteria can get trapped underneath the skin and sealed over.

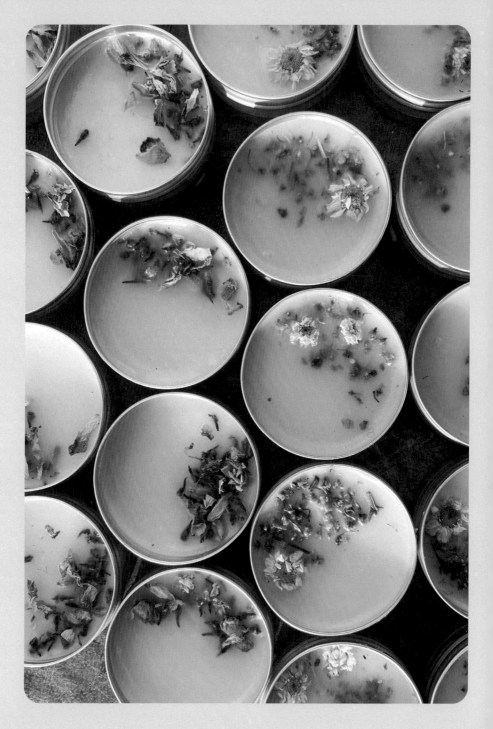

April

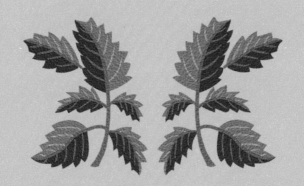

The spring showers and warmer temperatures bring with them a rush of new growth to the land. Warmer pockets are seeing a swift transformation, with hedgerows now clad in succulent growth. In contrast, the north experiences a slower unfolding of leaves and flowers, with branches often remaining bare and stubborn blossoms still reluctant to open.

Misty mornings bring about the sweet and heavy scent of honeysuckle while a sea of bluebells wash through the woodland. Out in the fields lie imperfect rings of lush green grass, forthcoming fungal clues to check back on later in the season. Nodding white flowers of three-cornered leek brighten up roadsides and shaded park corners; nestled in damp meadows the wild mints and meadowsweet grow taller; and a few cuckooflowers are just coming into bloom. Sap is rising in the trees, and there feels just enough sunshine to warm the cheeks.

Of course, April showers mean May flowers: gorse, lilacs and flowering currant all making delightfully refreshing syrups to preserve the flavours of spring. But showers also mean fungi! So, keep an eye out for St George's mushrooms towards the end of the month too.

Gorse

Ulex spp.

HARVEST TIME
All year-round
FAMILY
Fabaceae

A densely spiked evergreen shrub with cheerful yellow flowers known for their aromatic coconut scent, gorse can form impenetrable thickets, making them a valuable shelter for wildlife.

Recognizable by its tough, sharp, furrowed thorns with bright yellow, pea-like flowers that grow in clusters on three-angled branches. The coconut scent gets more intense in the warmer months and can be used as a natural navigation method, as flowers on the south side of the bush will have a stronger coconut flavour than those growing on the north. The texture of the flowers is also reminiscent of coconut.

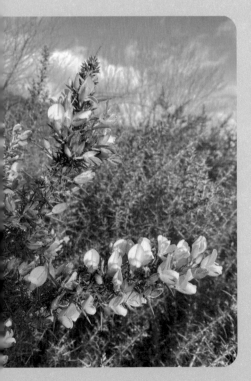

Traditionally, gorse has been used medicinally for its mild diuretic properties, to help treat digestive issues and as an antidote to melancholy. It can be used for weaving baskets and as a fuel for fires. The flowers can be used to make a fragrant tea, to help shift a glum mood.

Gorse is a perennial shrub with a few species, which extends the harvest time: common gorse (*Ulex europaeus*) flowers in the first six months of the year; with western gorse (*Ulex gallii*) and dwarf gorse (*Ulex minor*) flowering in the latter half of the year. All can be found in acidic environments, coastal areas, heathlands, meadows, open spaces and waste ground – don't forget your gloves!

LOOKALIKE: **Scotch broom**
(*Cytisus scoparius*)

Ground elder
Aegopodium podagraria

The arch nemesis of the gardener, ground elder is a hardy perennial that can have invasive tendencies, quickly carpeting damp, shady, nutrient-rich soils, lawns, woodlands and church grounds.

HARVEST TIME
Feb to May
FAMILY **Apiaceae**
COMMON NAMES
**Herb Gerard,
goutwort,
devil's guts**

Ground elder can be identified by its ovate/elliptical pointed leaves on short stalks, which are three-lobed with a serrated margin. Leaves look somewhat similar to the elder tree (*Sambucus nigra*), the explanation for its common name. In summer, upright, hairless grooved stems bear flat umbels of small white flowers.

Young leaves and stems can be eaten raw, and buttered ground elder shoots was a common medieval peasant dish. Flowers can be used as a garnish and the dried root ground into baking flour. Once the plant has flowered, usually in early spring, the taste changes dramatically, as do the medicinal qualities, causing the plant to have laxative effects. Ground elder has also been useful in helping to treat inflammation, rheumatic pains and insect bites.

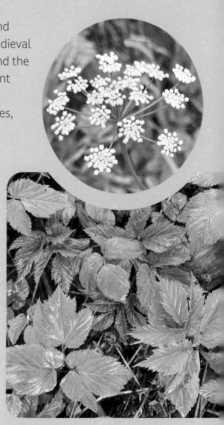

Spreading through rhizomes, ground elder can form dense ground cover. Be sure to collect only the youngest, freshest leaves for best flavour, as older leaves can leave you with a rather dreadful, lingering taste. The best time for harvesting is when the leaves are glossy, translucent and yet to unfurl – at this stage they have an inquisitive taste, somewhere between celery, carrot tops and aniseed.

LOOKALIKE:
💀 Dog's mercury (*Mercurialis perennis*)

Cleavers
Galium aparine

....

Caution
*Historically,
cleavers have been
used to prevent
pregnancies, so as a
precaution, avoid
using if pregnant or
breastfeeding.*

....

A scrambling herbaceous plant with clinging hairs on its stems, cleavers is known as a cleansing herb and is often found in hedgerows, gardens and waste areas.

Long, straggly, non-branching stems are covered in tiny hooked hairs that cling to surfaces and whorls of narrow leaves. In the summer, cleavers have tiny, star-shaped white flowers that morph into spherical seed burrs in autumn.

Hailed as a lymphatic tonic, cleavers enhance the function of the lymphatic system and improve the body's ability to flush out toxins. They can also help to protect the bladder lining and relieve an overactive bladder. A basic herbal infusion is perhaps one of the quickest and most effective ways to incorporate cleavers into your diet, or simply steep a big handful of cleavers in a jug of water and leave to infuse overnight.

Harvest young, tender tips for a subtle cucumber or pea shoot-like flavour when eaten fresh; they can also be cooked as a leafy green. The sticky leaves make for a great makeshift sieve, can be beaten to extract cordage fibres, and when dried becomes a flammable tinder material. Seed heads can be dried and ground into coffee, and a red dye can be extracted from the roots.

Cleavers can be found absolutely everywhere – gardens, woodlands, hedgerows, meadows and anywhere with well-watered, fertile soil.

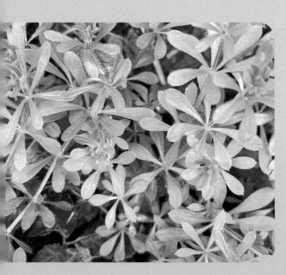

LOOKALIKE: **Bedstraw**
(*Galium* spp.)

Chickweed

Stellaria media

A delicate, creeping plant with small, oval leaves, chickweed can be eaten in place of spinach and even used as a moisturizer.

Identified by its sprawling and branching habit, stems are round with a single line of hair. Leaves grow in opposite pairs and are small, ovate to elliptical in shape, with tiny, star-shaped white flowers featuring five deeply notched petals.

Chickweed is a demulcent, meaning it can ease coughing and congestion in the lungs, help with inflammation and soothe the digestive tract. It can also be applied topically for skin conditions such as eczema, psoriasis, bites, stings and rashes. As a mucilage-rich herb, chickweed is a great moisturizer and can be used to make a cooling face mask: simply add a handful of fresh chickweed to a mortar and pestle along with two tablespoons of yoghurt; grind to a paste; and apply to clean, dry skin. To soothe itchy skin: blend together four parts chickweed to one part apple cider vinegar; strain through a muslin cloth; and add two tablespoons to your bath. Harvest young, tender leaves for salads, sandwiches and pesto, or cook and use in place of spinach.

Common chickweed can be found all year-round and prefers rich soil; look in gardens, cultivated fields and disturbed areas.

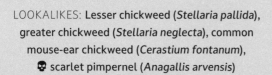

HARVEST TIME
All year-round
FAMILY
Caryophyllaceae
COMMON NAMES
**Birdweed,
starweed,
chickenwort**

LOOKALIKES: **Lesser chickweed (*Stellaria pallida*),
greater chickweed (*Stellaria neglecta*), common
mouse-ear chickweed (*Cerastium fontanum*),**
☠ **scarlet pimpernel (*Anagallis arvensis*)**

White dead nettle

Lamium album

HARVEST TIME
All year-round
FAMILY
Lamiaceae
COMMON NAME
White archangel

Looking like a stinging nettle before coming into flower, though unrelated, white dead nettle is devoid of stinging hairs and is actually a member of the mint family.

This common perennial, patch-forming plant is identified by its fibrous square stem, opposite heart-shaped leaves with fine, non-stinging hairs and toothed margins. Small hooded flowers form in circular clusters up the stem and are white with a hint of green on the lower lip, and have a black marking on the inside of the upper lip. White dead nettle blooms from March until November, or throughout winter in milder years.

White dead nettle tea has a mild sedative effect and is a helpful remedy for insomnia, digestive complaints and with regulating menstrual bleeding, while a cooled tea can be used as an eye wash or face tonic. Topical ointments soothe the skin and relieve menstrual cramps.

Leaves can be harvested throughout the year; when young, eat them fresh; for older leaves, cook as a spinach substitute. The flowers contain a sweet nectar that can be sucked directly from the tubular blossoms on a warm day, used as a garnish or dried for a medicinal tea. Dried leaves and flower stems can be preserved in vinegar or oil, whipped into a butter or blended into a powdered seasoning.

White dead nettle is frequently found in gardens, along hedgerows and fences, and in waste ground, churchyards and disturbed areas.

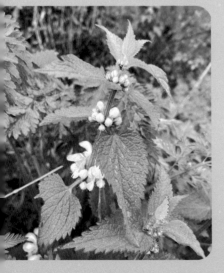

LOOKALIKES: Stinging nettle (*Urtica dioica*), red dead nettle (*Lamium purpureum*), yellow archangel (*Lamium galeobdolon*)

Red dead nettle
Lamium purpureum

An ideal plant to grow as ground cover in the garden, red dead nettle adds an attractive edible layer of protection to bare soil over winter, and is an awesome source of early nectar for bees.

This low-growing perennial has hairy, oval to heart-shaped green leaves, with a blunt serration or scalloped margin. Leaves grow in opposite pairs, are crowded along the square stem, are often tinged purple at the top of the plant and are stalked, unlike other dead nettles. Small, tubular pinkish-purple flowers are two-lipped and grow in whorls.

As an anti-inflammatory, anti-fungal and antibacterial plant, the leaves can be chewed to make a spit poultice for wounds and insect bites. Steep dried leaves for a tea, or infuse in oil for use in balms, salves and lotions. High in vitamins A, C and K, and rich in iron and fibre, red dead nettle is an immune-system ally. Make a tincture to help with inflammation and allergies by adding 50g (2oz) of dried dead nettle to 250ml (8fl oz) of high-proof alcohol, such as vodka, store somewhere dark for six weeks and shake every day. Take a few drops as needed. Eat leaves fresh when harvested young – they have an aromatic, peppery taste.

Common along woodland trails and in meadows, fields and waste ground, leaves grow year-round, with the plant blooming in all but the coldest of months.

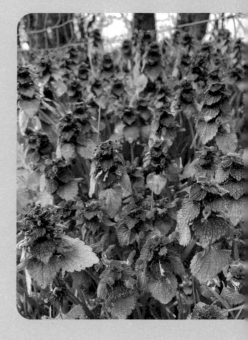

LOOKALIKES: **White dead nettle (*Lamium album*), stinging nettle (*Urtica dioica*), yellow archangel (*Lamium galeobdolon*)**

Morels

Morchella spp.

HARVEST TIME
Mar to May
FAMILY
Morchellaceae

A notoriously difficult group of mushrooms to find, don't let their elusive nature put you off: morels are worth the hunt. These highly sought-after gourmet mushrooms have a firm texture and nutty, earthy flavour.

Morels are typically around 5–12cm (2–4¾in) tall but can grow much larger. The cap colour varies from yellowish-brown to black, and it has a distinctive cone shape with a honeycomb-like pattern and deep pits or hollows, from which morels, being free of gills, release their spores. The cap and stem are joined together as a single piece: if you were to cut it open you would find a completely hollow interior – this is an important ID feature, and one that makes these great mushrooms into which to pipe a sauce!

Morels are a great source of iron and vitamin D. As an antioxidant, they can also help to strengthen the immune system. They must be cooked well before eating, and can be stored almost indefinitely when dried.

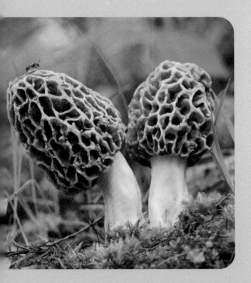

There are a number of closely related morel species, all of which are excellent edibles. The yellow morel (*Morchella esculenta*) and common morel (*Morchella vulgaris*) are said to grow in grassy patches of deciduous woodland areas and old orchards but are found more commonly in woodchip beds of public parks, estates and car parks, as is particularly the case for the compost-loving black morel (*Morchella importuna*).

LOOKALIKES:
☠ False morels (*Gyromitra* spp.), thimble morel (*Verpa conica*)

Pink purslane
Claytonia sibirica

This delicate herbaceous wildflower provides us with a spring green that is wholly edible, high in nutrients and provides a soothing, indulgent treat for the skin.

With a low-growing habit, pink purslane has both basal and flower leaves. Forming a rosette, the basal leaves are succulent, glossy and spoon-shaped or elliptical, while the flower leaves grow in opposite pairs, have no leaf stem and can appear joined at the base. The slender stems bear small star-shaped flowers with five deeply notched petals in varying shades of pink, often with darker pink veins, forming loose clusters that dangle atop opposite leaves.

High in mucilage, pink purslane acts as a natural demulcent and emollient, and is also high in vitamins A and C, phosphorus, calcium and iron. It can help to reduce inflammation, improve digestion and lower cholesterol levels. A fresh leaf poultice can be applied topically to rashes, bites and stings, or whipped into shea butter and coconut oil for an indulgent moisturizer. The fleshy leaves have an earthy, sometimes salty flavour, depending on habitat, and are perfect for bulking out salads; the flowers make for a pretty garnish.

Claytonia species are often found in meadows, fields, woodland edges and along stream banks.

HARVEST TIME
Mar to Aug
FAMILY
Montiaceae
COMMON NAME
Candy flower

Spring beauty (*Claytonia perfoliata*)
Similar to pink purslane, and used in the same way, spring beauty shares the low-growing, mat-forming rosette growth habit and fleshy, obovate-shaped leaves on long petioles. It can be distinguished by its tiny white flowers and fused, almost circular leaf that forms a cup around the flower stem.

Sweet violet
Viola odorata

HARVEST TIME
All year-round
FAMILY
Violaceae
COMMON NAME
Wood violet

A charming woodland wildflower giving flavour to those childhood-favourite sweets, Parma Violets, sweet violet is the only species of violet that is scented.

Sweet violets are low-growing perennial plants with crinkled, dark green, heart-shaped leaves with a serrated margin. Flowers are blueish to dark violet with a short, violet spur and blunt sepals. The flowers have five petals, with a larger lower petal that serves as a landing pad for pollinators.

Leaves are high in vitamins A and C, and are antioxidant and antiseptic. They contain salicylic acid and can be used topically as a fresh poultice to relieve pain and inflammation, extracted with an alcohol tincture to help break down warts, or made into tea by steeping the leaves in hot water as a soothing and tasty medicine for coughs, sore throats, respiratory ailments and menopause symptoms. Roots are diuretic, expectorant, emollient and cathartic, but should be used in moderation.

The leaves can be eaten raw in salads or cooked lightly as a spring green. Flowers are commonly crystallized in sugar for cake decorations at spring solstice celebrations. Make a deliciously fragrant syrup by steeping the flowers in a simple 1:1 sugar–water syrup in the fridge for 48 hours – it's pH reactive, so changes colour when you add lemon or tonic water. Harvest sustainably by taking only a single bloom from each plant. It is found in woodlands, hedgerows, shady meadows, grassy patches and gardens. Leaves can be found all year; the flowers bloom from March to June; harvest roots in autumn.

LOOKALIKES:
Other *Viola* spp.

Wild carrot
Daucus carota

Wild carrot is a delicate-looking but versatile and adaptable flowering plant with a characteristic seed head resembling a bird's nest, and it has been used traditionally as a carminative.

This branching biennial reaches 30–80cm (12–30in), with a hairy grooved stem, slender white taproot and feathery leaves with a mild, carroty aroma. Basal leaves form a rosette in the first year, while stem leaves are alternate, dissected and pinnately compound with a smooth upper surface and hairy underside. In its second year, wild carrot sends up a tall stem with multiple branches, each terminating in an umbel of tiny white flowers that have five petals, the central flower often red or dark purple. Umbels are surrounded by larger petal-like bracts. As the seeds mature, the umbel folds up. The seeds are ribbed, elongated and curved.

Wild carrot contains lots of vitamins (A, B and C), minerals and dietary fibre. It has diuretic properties, contains antioxidants that help neutralize free radicals, and has shown antibacterial activity against some pathogens.

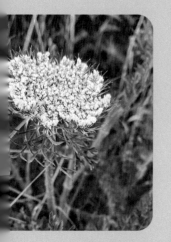

Use young leaves in salads or as a pot-herb. Roots have a more intense flavour – eat them fresh or try roasting and grinding into powder as a coffee alternative. Seeds can be dried and ground to produce an earthy spice.

Harvest leaves before the plant flowers around June; seeds in late summer to early autumn, when they have matured and turned brown; first-year roots in autumn, when less fibrous. Found in many habitats from meadows, roadsides and waste grounds to coastal areas.

HARVEST TIME
Apr to Nov
FAMILY
Apiaceae
COMMON NAMES
Queen Anne's lace,
bird's nest,
bishop's lace

Caution
*Wild carrot resembles the highly toxic poison hemlock (*Conium maculatum*) – see page 28. Extra caution must be taken in identifying members of the Apiaceae family. Also, if you have sensitive skin, contact with wild carrot can sometimes cause mild irritation.*

May

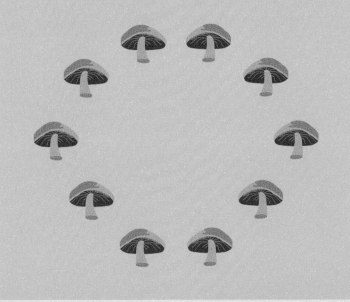

It could be one of life's sweetest treats to lie like a cat in the late spring sun beneath a big flowering hawthorn tree, getting just a little tipsy on the scent of its blossom.

Come May, all of the flowers seem in a hurry to open: oxeye daisies dance along motorway embankments; purple rock cress flows over garden walls like a tin of spilt paint; and the simple but pretty flowers of wild strawberries, raspberries, gooseberries and brambles are opening, some already bulging with next month's fruits.

The petals of wild cherry fall like confetti, and shards of sunlight pour in through unfurled leaves giving the bark a polished sheen. Yellow nuggets of chicken of the woods grow happily on their trunks, and ground elder now forms a mat on the forest floor below. Fiddlehead ferns push up their curled fronds and sweet woodruff sends up its flowers, ensuring as much light as possible before the canopy closes for the summer.

An hour's walk across the fields and through the woodland can easily fill a basket with salad greens of cleavers, chickweed, nettles and wild garlic; scented blooms of hawthorn, crab apple and cherry plum; and mushrooms such as the birch polypore, jelly ear and cauliflower fungus.

Nipplewort

Lapsana communis

HARVEST TIME
All year-round
FAMILY
Asteraceae

A tall, upright annual plant with a loosely branched, wiry appearance and flowers that look like miniature dandelions.

Identify nipplewort by its rosette of green, elongated alternate leaves that broaden with age, developing a rounded terminal lobe. Slender flower stems feature clusters of small compound flowers made up of yellow rayed florets and short outer bracts. The central stem is usually erect and hollow.

Flowers can be steeped in water to make a tea or can be boiled to extract a yellow dye; stems are fibrous and can be used to make paper, rope and cordage. Nipplewort has anti-inflammatory properties and the leaves can be used to treat skin conditions such as eczema and psoriasis, as well as cuts and burns. With a calming and antiseptic effect, nipplewort has been used as a herbal remedy for breast ulcers, cracked nipples and to staunch the flow of milk after breastfeeding, hence its name.

Harvest young and tender leaves for eating fresh – they have a slightly bitter taste and are similar to radish – or use the older leaves for cooking with. Nipplewort blooms between May and October, but the leaves are available year-round and are frequently found in gardens, cultivated fields, waste ground, gardens and disturbed soil.

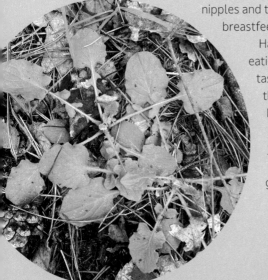

LOOKALIKES: **Prickly lettuce (*Lactuca serriola*), ragwort (*Senecio jacobaea*)**

Wood sorrel

Oxalis acetosella

With its mouth-wateringly zingy, citrus-like flavour, and the unmistakable heart-shaped leaves, wood sorrel is a good plant for first-time foragers: its lookalikes are edible too.

This low-growing, slow-creeping perennial has slightly hairy trifoliate leaves, each comprising of three heart-shaped leaflets and a central crease, enabling them to fold up at the end of the day. Open bell-shaped flowers are white, with pinkish-purple vein-like patterning on the inside of each of the five petals. Cylindrical exploding pods disperse seed several metres into the air.

Wood sorrel is rich in vitamin C and was once used to treat scurvy; it is also high in iron, potassium and fibre, and can be used to help calm an upset stomach and support liver health. It has also been used as a folk remedy to cure the hiccups. The leaves and flowers have a pleasantly sharp, acidic taste similar to tart apple peel, and they are best added to salads, stirred into a palate-cleansing sorbet, or just eaten fresh on the trail.

Wood sorrel can be found all year-round, but the flowers appear from late March and are often gone by July.

HARVEST TIME
All year-round
FAMILY
Oxalidaceae
COMMON NAMES
Wood sour, sour grass, fairy bells

Caution
As with the similarly tasting sheep sorrel and common sorrel, wood sorrel contains oxalic acid, so take care if you suffer from gout, arthritis or kidney stones.

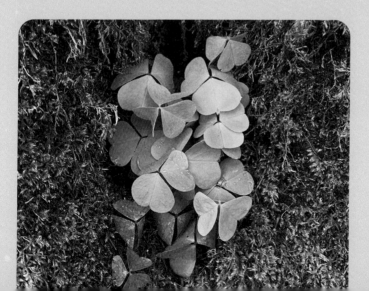

LOOKALIKES:
Black medic (*Medicago lupulina*), clover (*Trifolium*), other *Oxalis* spp.

St George's mushroom
Calocybe gambosa

HARVEST TIME
Apr to June
FAMILY
Lyophyllaceae
COMMON NAME
May mushroom
SPORE PRINT
White

Generally easy to identify due to their growing season, habitat and distinctive scent, these stocky white mushrooms are often found growing in fairy rings around St George's Day (23rd April), hence their name.

The white, domed, in-rolled cap can grow from 5–15cm (2–6in) in diameter, starting off convex and becoming flat, sometimes discolouring to a buff tan in older or damaged mushrooms. White gills are narrow, densely crowded and have a sinuate attachment. The firm and chunky white stem is around 2–8cm (¾–3in) tall and has no annulus (ring) but is often curving with a slightly swollen or bulbous base.

Containing vitamins B and D, St George's mushrooms are also known to help reduce blood sugar levels, so could be a helpful addition to a diet for diabetes.

St George's mushrooms are described as having a farinaceous, or 'mealy', aroma, often likened to freshly ground flour, wet dough, cucumber or watermelon rind. They are awesome sautéed or stir fried, and the meaty texture makes them good candidates for preserving.

Find these mushrooms in grassy areas – verges, meadows, fields lawns and woodland edges – in April and May, sometimes into mid-June.

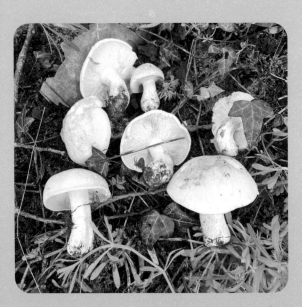

LOOKALIKES:
☠ **Deadly fibrecap**
(*Inocybe erubescens*),
miller mushroom
(*Clitopilus prunulus*)

Dryad's saddle
Polyporus squamosus

Dryad's saddle is a huge, almost circular bracket mushroom with distinctive brown concentric 'feathers', or scales, on the cap surface, earning its other popular common name of pheasant's back mushroom and making it difficult to confuse with any other mushroom.

HARVEST TIME
Apr to Aug
FAMILY
Polyporaceae
COMMON NAMES
Pheasant's back
mushroom,
scaly polypore
SPORE PRINT
White

As a polypore, you won't find gills underneath this mushroom, but instead large, irregularly shaped pores that start an off-white colour, yellowing with age. Though a bracket mushroom, you'll often find a large thick stipe connecting the cap to the tree; the stipe will often crack and fissure with age. Slicing the flesh reveals a fresh scent reminiscent of watermelon rind, which turns into a more savoury mushroomy smell once dried or cooked.

When harvesting, be sure to select young, flexible caps, as they tend to toughen as they grow. You can slice off the softer perimeter pieces of larger mushrooms. Peeling the top 'skin' from the cap before cooking can also help to make them more tender. Use as a pizza topping, along with wild garlic seed heads and purple rock cress flowers, which are also in season.

Found on decaying hardwoods, particularly oak trees in spring and early summer. You can often find dryad's saddle on the floor beneath its tree host, toppled over under its own weight.

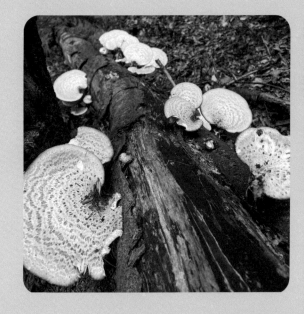

Stitchwort

Stellaria spp.

HARVEST TIME
Apr to June
FAMILY
Caryophyllaceae

These delicate herbaceous plants have small, star-shaped flowers, and the name 'stitchwort' is believed to have originated from the plant's historical use in treating the pain you get in your side after strenuous sporting activity – or an over-enthusiastic forage.

The flowers have five deeply divided petals, giving them a star-like appearance. Greyish-green sessile leaves are typically narrow, growing in opposite pairs on a fragile stem. Seed heads have an audible pop when mature or stepped on.

Stitchwort is useful as a salve or cream for the treatment of skin conditions such as eczema, psoriasis, insect bites and rashes. A compress can be made to help heal broken and fractured bones, and the plant is currently being tested for the treatment of sepsis and organ transplants.

As a food source, stitchwort is high in vitamins A, B12, C and D, as well as potassium, iron, zinc, calcium and silica. Use leaves and shoots in salads, or steamed or boiled as a spring green. Flowers can be used as a decorative garnish.

Greater stitchwort (*Stellaria holostea*) is found in damp, shady areas of grassland and in woodland edges. Lesser stitchwort (*Stellaria graminea*) is often found in fields and meadows, and, as the name would suggest, marsh stitchwort (*Stellaria palustris*) can be found in bogs, marshes and wetlands. Stitchwort blooms in spring and early summer.

LOOKALIKE: Chickweed (*Stellaria media*)

Purple rock cress
Aubrieta deltoidea

Purple rock cress is that vivid purple plant you see cascading over walls at this time of year, almost looking like someone has spilt a tin of paint. It has the typically cress-like peppery flavour.

This plant is a low-growing perennial with evergreen foliage and a trailing or procumbent growth habit. Trailing stems bear small, spoon-shaped to obovate leaves that are alternate on the stem, hairy and often displaying a serrated margin. *Aubrieta* produces terminal clusters of small four-petalled cruciform flowers from early April to July, often in vibrant shades of purple, pink and occasionally white. The flowers develop into slender, cylindrical seed pods known as siliques.

   Purple rock cress is a part of the Brassicaceae family of plants known to prevent oxidative stress and stimulate the immune system. All parts of the plant are edible: the flowers can be added to salads or sandwiches and have a mildly peppery flavour; the leaves can be used as a pot-herb.

   Both drought- and low-temperature tolerant, purple rock cress can be found on walls and rocky slopes, and on free-draining or stony sites. Spreading rapidly, it is often grown as a pollinator-friendly groundcover in gardens.

HARVEST TIME
Apr to July
FAMILY
Brassicaceae
COMMON NAMES
Devil's ivy, rainbow rock cress

Interesting fact
Aubrieta, *the genus name for purple rock cress, honours Claude Aubriet (1665–1742), a French botanical artist.*

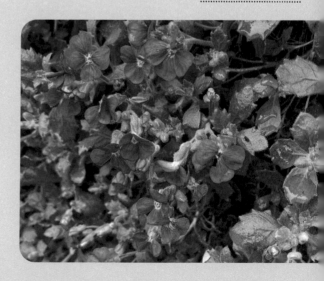

LOOKALIKES:
Bellflower (Campanula spp.), other *Aubrieta* spp.

Cuckooflower
Cardamine pratensis

HARVEST TIME
Apr to Aug
FAMILY
Brassicaceae
COMMON NAMES
**Lady's smock,
milkmaids**

These small, delicate wildflowers beckon the arrival of spring and the call of the cuckoo bird.

Upright spikes of narrow-stalked flowers in shades of pink or lilac (sometimes white) have four notched, overlapping petals with dark pink veins forming captivating patterns. The flowers have yellow anthers, and the basal rosettes sport pinnate leaves with a larger terminal leaflet.

Cuckooflower is antibacterial, antiviral and antioxidant, as well as having a high vitamin content which meant it was a popular prescription for scurvy. The leaves have hints of watercress flavour and have traditionally been used as a digestive to help prevent indigestion and promote appetite. Seeds and flowers have a sweet and spicy kick and can be dried for use as a seasoning.

Find this plant in damp meadows, pond margins, stream edges and riverbanks, with flowers arriving in April and peaking during May and early June.

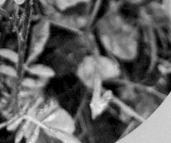

LOOKALIKES:
**Greater cuckooflower
(*Cardamine raphanifolia*), wavy bittercress
(*Cardamine flexuosa*)**

Oxeye daisy
Leucanthemum vulgare

Those giant daisies you see growing on the verges when you're driving along the motorway are oxeye daisies – pretty, perennial plants with an aromatic, herby flavour.

Growing on tall stems up to 1½m (5ft), this clump-forming plant starts as a basal rosette of spoon-shaped, scalloped leaves with a rounded, irregular serration. White petals surround yellow-centred disc-shaped flowers.

Oxeye daisy is a tonic herb helping to support overall well-being. Related to the arnica flower, the leaves and flowers share similar healing properties and can be infused into a carrier oil to make a skin-soothing, inflammation-fighting salve. A tea from the leaves and flowers can be taken to help promote collagen production, while the cooled tea makes a soothing topical face toner. The flowers and leaves can be used in salads, and the tight, unopened flower buds pickled like capers.

With invasive tendencies that see it quickly cover huge patches of grass or bare soil with its creeping rhizomes, you'll find oxeye in meadows, field edges, roadside verges and disturbed areas. It blooms from April through to August.

HARVEST TIME
Apr to Aug
FAMILY
Asteraceae
COMMON NAMES
Marguerite, moon
daisy, dog daisy

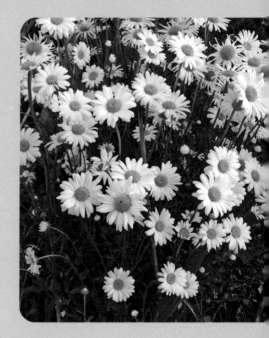

LOOKALIKES:
Shasta daisy (*Leucanthemum* x *superbum*),
common daisy (*Bellis perennis*)

Linden tree
Tilia spp.

HARVEST TIME
May to Sept
FAMILY
Malvaceae
COMMON NAME
Lime tree

Growing up to 45m (148ft) tall, these deciduous 'street trees' are known for their fragrant flowers and large, heart-shaped leaves. This is a tree you can identify from a distance due to the 'suckers' at its base or middle.

The smooth grey-brown bark of the *Linden* flakes as it matures. The leaves can grow up to 10cm (4in) and are asymmetrical with a coarsely serrated leaf margin. They are often covered in a sticky honeydew, making them sweet, for a leaf. Clusters of five-petalled green-yellow flowers hang from a leaf bract.

The flowers have a naturally sweet, floral flavour and can be used to make a hydrating tea that soothes digestion, fights inflammation and calms anxiety. *Linden* leaves and flowers act as a vasodilator, widening the blood vessels and lowering blood pressure. Flowers and bracts have also been dried and smoked as a tobacco alternative, and to help with clarity and focus.

Leaves can be harvested all summer but are best when still young and translucent. Catch them before they start to unfurl in April and May for a taste similar to sugar snap peas; larger leaves make good dolma wraps. The oval seed pods are also edible and many claim they can be a chocolate substitute.

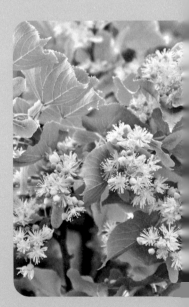

Mostly found in parks and gardens, often planted in villages, towns and cities as shade trees and as a bioremediatory, *Lindens* flower between May and July.

Interesting fact
Linden *trees can help draw and trap toxins from the air through their leaves, which means you should be especially fastidious about where you choose to forage your* Linden *leaves!*

Pineappleweed
Matricaria discoidea

This underrated plant has a truly tropical aroma, one that always astounds with its strong pineapple scent and fruity flavour. The low-growing, branching herb lacks an important feature you'd normally expect from a flower – petals!

HARVEST TIME
Feb to Nov
FAMILY
Asteraceae
COMMON NAMES
Wild chamomile,
disc mayweed,
rayless mayweed

Conical, dome-shaped button heads of yellow disc-shaped florets with green bracts emit a sweet, fruity, citrusy scent when crushed, similar to chamomile. The heads sit above rosettes of wispy, deeply lobed, fern-like leaves that grow in an alternate arrangement on the stem. Once mature, the plant develops brown achenes that each contain a seed, with one head holding as many as 500.

Pineappleweed imparts a sedative effect, helping to stem restlessness and promote sleep. Traditionally used as a cleansing tea for worms and parasites, the leaves and heads can also be crushed and rubbed onto the skin as an insect repellent, or added to a high-proof alcohol to create a skin-healing tincture for use in salves, balms, lotions and toners. Make into a syrup to top yoghurt or liven up a cocktail; combine with oil and vinegar for a salad dressing; or eat fresh and raw for a nutrient-rich, energy-boosting trail snack. Leaves have a mildly bitter, grass-like flavour.

Established pineappleweed grows new leaves from February, and lies almost undetected until it starts to 'flower' from April. There's a second flush in the autumn from spring-grown plants. From arable fields to wasteland, gardens to allotment lanes and roadside verges, pineappleweed thrives in compacted soils, so you're also likely to find it on a well-trodden grassy path.

LOOKALIKES: **Scented mayweed (*Matricaria chamomilla*), field chamomile (*Anthemis arvensis*)**

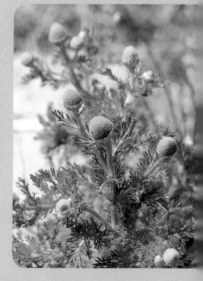

Scurvy grass
Cochlearia officinalis

HARVEST TIME
Mar to Oct
FAMILY
Brassicaceae
COMMON NAMES
Spoonwort,
scrubbyweed

Scurvy grass is a peppery, coastal plant with small, spoon-shaped leaves. It was historically consumed to prevent scurvy due to being an easily accessible source of vitamin C.

A low-growing plant with rosettes of glossy, spoon-, heart- or kidney-shaped leaves between 1–6cm (½–2¼in) in diameter, with prominent veins. Upper leaves are sessile; lower leaves are stalked; and it has clusters of small white flowers.

As well as its documented use among sailors, scurvy grass is considered to be an effective blood purifier, and it is recommended to be blended and drank as a juice shot each morning – though I can think of a hundred more plants I'd

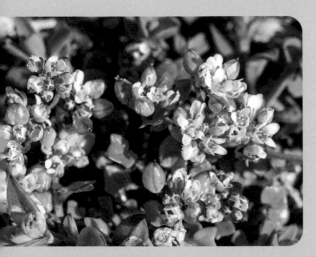

sooner drink than scurvy grass! Leaves are at their most pungent during the spring and summer months; the strong flavour is certainly not to everyone's liking, but it does become milder as the season goes on. Try using in sushi for a local wasabi flavour, or drying and powdering for a seasoning. The flowers, however, are an awesome garnish sprinkled over salads. If you are a fan of bitter, horseradish-like heat, then try popping an unripe green seed pod in your mouth – succulent and crunchy, but very pungent! Found on coastal cliffs, salt marshes and along seashores from March until October.

LOOKALIKE: **Lesser celandine (*Ficaria verna*)**

Elm tree

Ulmus spp.

Elms are deciduous trees, with a vase-like shape, able to grow over 18m (60ft) tall. There are more than 30 species, but many share common features.

HARVEST TIME
All year-round
FAMILY
Ulmaceae

Look for green, doubly serrated leaves, often asymmetrical at the base and turning yellow in autumn. The grey-brown bark is deeply ridged, and reddish-pink flowers bloom in clusters before the leaves emerge. The edible fruits, known as samaras, start out like a leaf before growing a seed in the centre, developing an oiliness once mature, before turning brittle and brown, ready to fall and be dispersed by the wind.

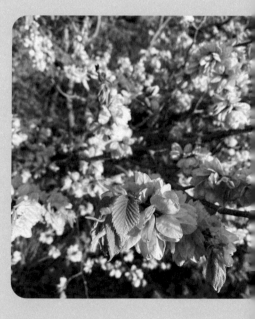

The bark can be dried and powdered to be made into a soothing tea for sore throats, boiled with milk for a bone-healing porridge, or mixed with honey and water to form throat-coating cough drops. Mucilaginous leaves are antiseptic; use as a fresh poultice or tea.

Add samaras to salads or eat as a trail snack while out foraging, although they are tough once the casing becomes brown and papery. The seeds can also be eaten and have a nutty flavour; remove the paper casing and use as you would sunflower seeds. Dry, grind and mix the inner bark with butter to form a roux for thickening soups and stews.

Harvest samaras from April when they are green and tender; leaves when they first appear around May; the inner bark all year-round. Elms are found in a variety of habitats, from forests to cities, often planted as shade trees in parks and urban areas.

Lilacs

Syringa spp.

HARVEST TIME
May & June
FAMILY
Oleaceae

As a colourful, fragrant flower, lilacs are often used to impart a delicate floral flavour to desserts and baked goods, and make for a pretty, edible garnish.

The broad, simple leaves are dark green and heart shaped. Spikes of tiny, densely packed tubular flowers in shades of lilac, pink and sometimes white, grow in large cone-shaped clusters called racemes. Typically grows to 6m (20ft) tall.

Lilac stimulates the digestive tract, helping to aid digestion and reduce bloating. Infused lilac water can be used as a topical astringent to help soothe and tone irritated skin, and relieve insect bites, minor burns and rashes. Harvest lilac with newly opened blooms for the most flavour. Steep blossoms in honey for a floral sweetener; infuse into alcohol, or milk and sugar, for use in baked goods; or use the flowers to make jelly, wine and ice cream.

Lilacs are often found in parks and gardens, where certain species are planted as hedging.

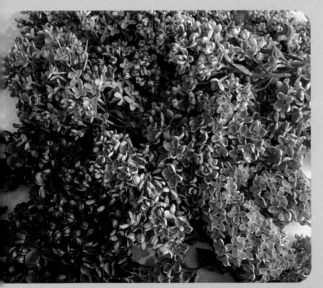

LOOKALIKES:
Butterfly bush (*buddleja* spp.)

Lilac syrup

One of the most popular ways to utilize lilac is to make a versatile syrup. I have made a lot of flower syrups over the years, but the first I ever made was with lilac flowers from the towering, unruly shrub of my childhood back garden. I have been experimenting with infusion times ever since, and this is my favourite recipe for retaining the delicate flavour that can often be lost in the process.

Once made, the syrup can be drizzled over ice cream, waffles or pancakes; mixed with homemade lemonade and frozen into lolly moulds; stirred into hot chocolate; or brushed onto cakes to keep them moist.

3 lilac racemes
250ml (1 cup) water
150ml (5fl oz) honey
Sterilized bottles/ice
    cube trays

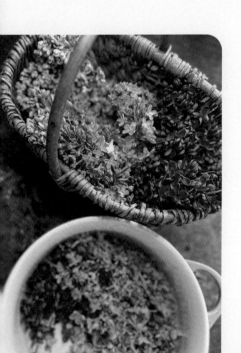

1. Carefully pull the individual flowers from three lilac racemes – a little patience pays here, as too many green stems will make your syrup bitter.

2. Add the flowers to the water.

3. Cover, and steep in the fridge for 24–48 hours – the longer, the stronger.

4. Once strained, stir in the honey.

5. Decant into sterilized bottles to keep in the fridge for use over a week or two, or freeze in ice cube trays for quick lemonades and cocktails.

Field mint
Mentha arvensis

HARVEST TIME
Apr to Oct
FAMILY
Lamiaceae
COMMON NAMES
Wild mint,
corn mint

Field mint grows abundantly in a diverse array of habitats, and is known for its digestive properties. The plant has a strong, pleasant minty aroma when crushed and can be used in the same way as cultivated mint.

Field mint is a perennial herb reaching 10–60cm (4–24in), but often taller. It has a branching habit with erect or semi-sprawling square stems and simple, hairy leaves found in opposing pairs and displaying a coarsely serrated margin. Whorls of tiny, delicate tubular flowers form clusters at the stem bases. Flowers appear between June and September, and are most often pale purple, but sometimes white or pink. The fruit that follows is a two-chambered carpel.

One key component of field mint is menthol, which has a soothing effect on the muscles of the digestive tract. The plant also contains volatile oils such as menthone and limonene, which not only contribute to its aromatic profile, but also have carminative properties, helping to alleviate gas and bloating.

Young top shoots provide the most intense flavour. Make a classic mint sauce by blitzing a large handful of foraged mint with 1 teaspoon of sugar and 3 tablespoons of white wine vinegar. Or make a mint chocolate-chip ice cream by blending mint leaves, coconut milk, nut butter and maple syrup, or birch syrup, together; freeze in an ice cube tray, then transfer to a food processor; add chocolate chunks and blitz until you reach a soft-serve consistency.

Field mint can be found in fields, meadows, pastures, farm borders and as an escapee outside allotment lanes. Gathering stems on a dry day after the morning dew has evaporated will help prevent leaves from turning black when drying.

LOOKALIKES
**Water mint
(*Mentha aquatica*),
spearmint
(*Mentha spicata*),
peppermint
(*Mentha × piperita*)**

Sea kale

Crambe maritima

The best time to harvest this coastal plant is in spring, before it starts to flower and while the young, unfolding shoots are still tender. Sea kale tastes like a cross between celery and asparagus.

The thick, fleshy leaves form low-growing clumps, reaching 30–60cm (12–24in). They emerge purple, turning bluish green as they grow, and become fleshy, lobed or pinnately divided, with an entire or crinkled margin. The stems are smooth and stout, and the leaves have a distinctive, often clasping or semi-amplexicaul base, partially encircling the stem. Small, white, fragrant flowers have four overlapping petals and are arranged in dense terminal clusters, blooming in late spring to early summer. Round, green seed pods appear after flowering, containing small, peppery seeds.

HARVEST TIME
Mar to Oct
FAMILY
Brassicaceae
COMMON NAME
Sea cabbage

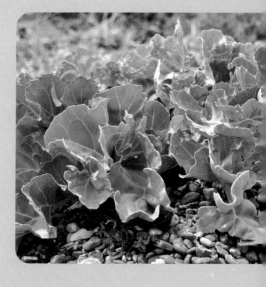

A good source of vitamins C and A, calcium, potassium, magnesium and dietary fibre, sea kale is also an antioxidant and anti-inflammatory. Leaves can be applied topically to aid in wound healing. The young shoots can be eaten raw in salads; shredded and cooked like cabbage by steaming, boiling or sautéing; or used to add flavour and texture to soups and quiches. The flowers have a milder flavour and can be used as a garnish. Seed pods can be pickled, or the inside seeds ground into a powder and used as a condiment or spice.

Commonly found in coastal areas, especially on shingle beaches, sand dunes and sandy or well-draining soils.

LOOKALIKE
Sea beet (*Beta vulgaris maritima*)

June

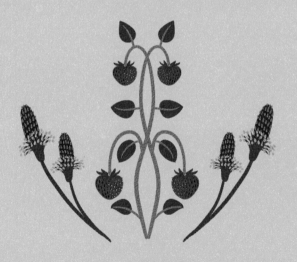

June heralds the start of peak wild swimming season, and it's when bodies of water are particularly rich in interesting plant life and buoyant with bloom: from marsh marigolds to angelica, bull rush, skullcap and pendulous sedge. Freshly plucked wild radish seed pods add some heat to summer picnics, and the sweet nectar sipped straight from dead nettle flowers is not to be missed on a sunny day.

Fluffy heads of salsify catch the wind and float through blue skies, it's air filled with the sweet fragrance of dog rose. Towering spikes of yellow flowers are sent up from the fuzzy pale green basal leaves of mullein, and tall purple plumes of loosestrife watch over water lilies floating on the glassy lake, while effervescent dragonflies dart above its surface.

One really doesn't need to go far to find an abundance of wild food this month – a typical small lawn or 'weedy' patio garden can contain as many as a hundred or more edible plants throughout the year. Broadleaf and ribwort plantain, clover, vetch, wood avens, dandelion, sorrel – the list is longer than these pages have room for.

Common elder

Sambucus nigra

HARVEST TIME
May to Sept
FAMILY
Adoxaceae
COMMON NAME
Elderberry

The frothy, creamy white flowers of the elder tree or shrub are a common sight and scent of the countryside, marking the start of summer, when they can be collected for best flavour.

Compound and pinnate leaves are comprised of five or seven toothed leaflets arranged in opposite pairs, with a terminal toothed leaflet. Young twigs are green, brittle and contain a white pith, turning grey or pale brown. Mature bark is furrowed and corky. From late May until mid-June, tiny clusters of tight green buds open up into scented white flowers, growing at the end of florets and forming large heads, or 'sprays'.

Flowers steeped in water can be used as a treatment for sunburn, shaving rash and blemishes. Elderflower water can be used as a mosquito repellent and as a compress for tired eyes. Leaves are toxic when eaten but can be used to make green elder ointment, to help treat aches, sprains and bruises, and to create a protective barrier and moisturize the skin. The flowers are turned into syrups, cordials and 'champagne', but can also be used to flavour jams and jellies, and they make a delicious floral-tasting vinegar, too. Gather just-opened clusters of blooms on a warm, dry morning for best flavour – if it is sunny, keep an eye out for bugs hiding inside. Do not rinse, as this will remove the fragrant pollen. At the end of summer, elder provides deep purple berries that are high in fibre and full of vitamin C and antioxidants. While toxic raw, when cooked they make a tasty immune-boosting syrup that will ward off winter illness.

LOOKALIKE: **Dwarf elder (*Sambucus ebulus*)**

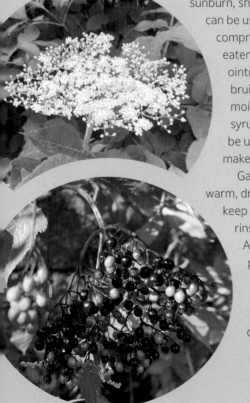

Sea purslane
Halimione portulacoides

A low-growing, sprawling perennial shrub, sea purslane's silvery, salty, succulent leaves have a thick, crunchy texture.

HARVEST TIME
Apr to Aug
FAMILY
Amaranthaceae

The fleshy, silver-green leaves are oval or linear to lanceolate, with a full margin and sometimes a red or pink blush at the tips. The opposite leaves grow on smooth stems that become tough and woody as the plant matures. The wind-pollinated flowers are small and yellow, with five petals, and appear on slender spikes or clusters.

Halophytes (salt-tolerant plants) have a richer mineral content than other edible plants, and sea purslane in particular contains high levels of sodium, potassium, calcium, magnesium and phosphorus, and is also high in omega 3 fatty acids. After a good rinse to remove any mud or sand, the leaves can be eaten fresh in salads or sandwiches, cooked into dishes, added to pickle jars, or dried and powdered for a salt substitute – especially good whipped through homemade butter. Flower buds can be preserved in vinegar, similar to capers, or opened flowers used as a garnish.

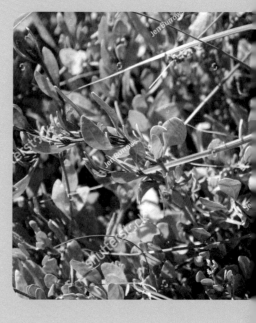

As a phytoremediator, sea purslane is often planted around polluted coastlines to help remove heavy metals and toxins from contaminated soil (around 90 per cent of these are stored in its deep root system). It is at its most succulent from April through to August; however, as an evergreen plant, you will find it growing all year-round on saltmarshes, estuaries and sandy or muddy coastlines.

Elderberry lollipops

Not only do these two-ingredient homemade lollipops offer a fun treat, but they also harness the immune-boosting prowess of elderberries, complemented by the soothing touch of honey – a sweet remedy for sore or scratchy throats.

If you don't have a jam thermometer, pop a little mixture into a cold glass of water and if it turns hard, it's ready. And if you don't have lollipop mould, just pour careful dollops onto a sheet of baking paper.

To make approx 500ml (2 cups):
250g (9oz) ripe elderberries
200g (7oz) honey or sugar
Optional spices: e.g. chopped sweet cicely or wood avens root, sumac or dried magnolia petals

To make the elderberry syrup:

1. Harvest the heads of ripe elderberries and use a fork to strip the berries from their stems.

2. Place the berries (and any optional extras) into a saucepan and add water until they are just submerged.

3. Bring to the boil, then turn down the heat and simmer gently until the berries burst open.

4. Once cooled, sieve the mixture through a fine mesh. You can use this juice as is for cooking or baking.

5. To turn the juice into a syrup for your lollipops, pour the honey or sugar and elderberry juice into a saucepan and bring to a simmer until everything has dissolved.

6. Once cooled, bottle and store in the fridge or freezer.

To make the lollipops:

200ml (1 cup) elderberry syrup
100g (3½oz) honey

1. In a small saucepan, combine the elderberry syrup and honey over a low heat.

2. Stir the mixture continuously, until the honey has melted and combined.

3. Increase the heat to medium and clip a jam thermometer in the pot.

4. Continue stirring every now and then until it reaches a temperature of 150°C (302°F). This is known as the 'hard ball' stage.

5. Remove the saucepan from the heat and let it cool for a few minutes before pouring into your lolly moulds and popping in your sticks.

6. Sprinkle with dried elderflower and leave to set in the fridge.

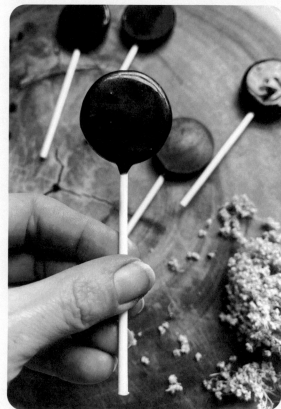

Store your lollipops in a sealed jar; I roll mine in powdered sugar to prevent them sticking together.

Wild strawberry

Fragaria vesca

HARVEST TIME
May to Sept
FAMILY **Rosaceae**
COMMON NAMES
**Woodland
strawberry,
Alpine strawberry**

Much tastier than cultivated strawberries, wild strawberries, with their almost artificial sweetness, are a true summer delight.

Identification of wild strawberries is easy, as they look just like our cultivated garden strawberries, only much daintier. They have three lobed, deeply crimped, shiny, serrated leaves and hairy flower stems bearing small white flowers with five slightly overlapping petals. A perennial plant that spreads via runners, it can cover large patches of ground in just a few years.

Crushed berries can help relieve sunburn, and a strong tea made from the leaves can be used to treat a sore throat. The entire plant is edible, with the leaves and roots being high in tannins and the berries full of vitamin C, antioxidants and anti-inflammatory terpenes.

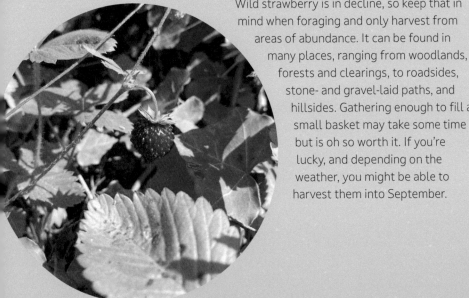

Wild strawberry is in decline, so keep that in mind when foraging and only harvest from areas of abundance. It can be found in many places, ranging from woodlands, forests and clearings, to roadsides, stone- and gravel-laid paths, and hillsides. Gathering enough to fill a small basket may take some time but is oh so worth it. If you're lucky, and depending on the weather, you might be able to harvest them into September.

LOOKALIKE: **Barren strawberry (*Potentilla sterilis*)**

Motherwort

Leonurus cardiaca

The tall motherwort, known as the 'mother plant', is noted for supporting female health and fertility.

Motherwort typically reaches heights of 50–120cm (2–4ft). It has a heavily ridged square stem; opposite palmate leaves, the same colour on both sides, with three to five sharply pointed lobes attached by long petioles; and whirls of small tubular flowers divided into two lips, which can be white, pale pink or pale purple.

Renowned for its anti-inflammatory and anti-microbial properties, it is used as a uterine tonic, eases cramps, regulates menstrual cycles, prevents blood clots, and aids in labour. Additionally, motherwort is a trusted remedy for reducing stress and enhancing mood. Thanks in part to the primary active alkaloid, leonurine, it is also suitable as a cardiotonic.

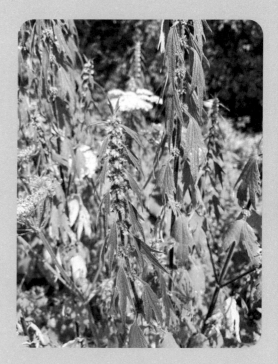

Motherwort has a pungent flavour, so is best prepared as a blend for teas or tinctures. Aside from traditional medicinal uses, it is also a flavourful addition to soups, teas and even beer.

Harvest motherwort when it comes into bloom, but be mindful when harvesting as wild populations appear to be on the decrease and are often scattered or localized. You will normally find this plant on waste ground or at roadsides.

LOOKALIKE: **Mugwort (*Artemisia vulgaris*)**

Red clover
Trifolium pratense

An easy plant to identify, with its three (or four, if you're lucky!) rounded leaves, red clover is full of essential vitamins and minerals, and all parts are edible.

Each of the leaves of red clover has a white crescent or V-shaped marking, and the plant bears tall, dark pinkish-red, fluffy, pompom-like flower heads.

A soothing plant for menstruation, extracts and tinctures can help treat symptoms of menopause, ease hot flushes, and calm and relax the body. Red clover is high in isoflavones (oestrogen-imitating chemicals), which can help relieve hormonal symptoms around ovulation, and is also said to aid treatment of osteoporosis in post-menopausal women.

Being a member of the Pea family, the plant has a hint of pea to its taste. Use the leaves in salads, infuse flowers into vodka or vinegar, or make a refreshing flower iced tea. Dried flowers can also be pounded into a gluten-free baking flour.

You'll find this plant growing in fields, meadows, parks and gardens. Harvest the leaves all year-round, the flowers from May to October.

LOOKALIKES: **White clover (*Trifolium repens*), wood sorrel (*Oxalis acetosella*)**

Dog rose
Rosa canina

From the fragrant summertime flowers to the plump autumnal rosehips, dog rose offers beauty, flavour, nutritional benefits and medicinal value.

HARVEST TIME
June to Nov
FAMILY
Rosaceae
COMMON NAME
Witches' briar

Come summertime, this perennial climbing shrub is covered in flowers of various shades of pink. The flowers have multiple uses and can be: eaten fresh as a garnish to salads; dried and crumbled onto desserts; candied and preserved; used to flavour jams, jellies, syrups and pastries; dried and blended into sugar to garnish cocktail rims; and even made into wine.

In autumn the flowers turn into edible seed pods that, when fully ripe and slightly bletted, become a delicious, sweet, tart flavour, and a fibrous, mushy texture, so they are best picked after the first frost. Full of antioxidants, they help to boost the immune system and protect against heart disease. Rosehips are so high in vitamin C that they actually led to its discovery. They can be turned into wine, jams, preserved in sugar or honey, or simply dried and made into tea.

Be aware that the seeds inside the fruits are covered in fine hairs that can irritate the skin, mouth and throat, and so need to be scraped out before eating. Pass cooked or blended fruits for syrups, jams or juices through a double layer of tight muslin cloth to remove the hairs.

As all rosehips are edible, this is a safe plant to forage, as long as it's not in or near an area that's been sprayed with chemicals.

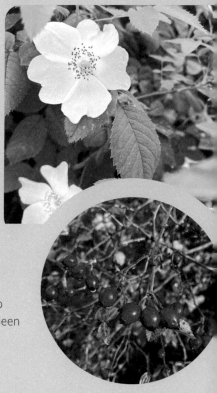

LOOKALIKES:
All species of rose

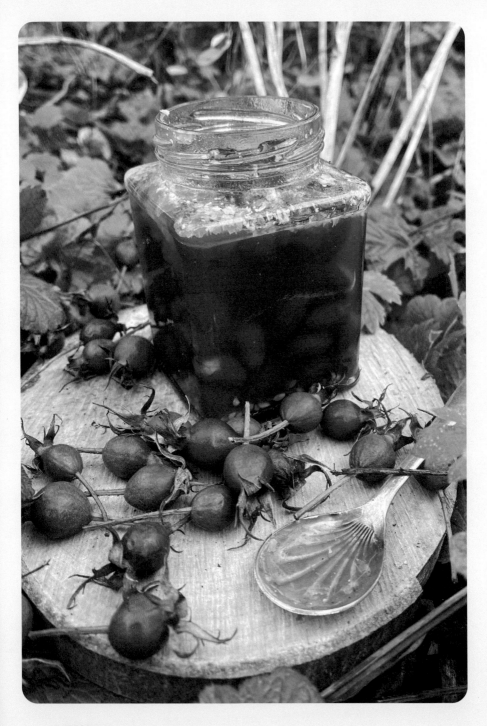

Rosehip oxymel

An oxymel is a sweet and tangy herbal remedy made by combining vinegar (often apple cider vinegar) and honey, along with your chosen herbs or fruits – in this case, vitamin C-rich rosehips.

Oxymel has a shelf life of around a year. Take it neat by the spoonful when you feel signs of sickness, or dilute into a glass of water and take daily as a preventative measure, or to stimulate metabolism in the morning. Rosehip oxymel can also be used as a salad dressing or marinade, and to clean wounds and treat infections. Rosehips are best harvested after a frost so they are softened.

Large handful of rosehips
Unpasteurized cider
   vinegar (with the lively
   mother still in)
Generous dollop of
   local honey
Optional spices: common
   hogweed seed,
   angelica seed, etc.

1. Prepare your rosehips by double-straining them through a fine mesh to remove the hairs. Roughly chop them and place in a sterilized jar.

2. Pour over the cider vinegar, ensuring it blankets the rosehips and leaves an inch or so on top.

3. Add any spices that you fancy.

4. Sweeten with local honey for the perfect oxymel balance.

Rosehips are abundant in vitamin C; however, high temperatures during cooking can lead to the breakdown of vitamin C molecules, reducing their effectiveness. By not cooking the rosehips in this recipe, the vitamin C content is preserved, ensuring the resulting oxymel retains its immune-boosting benefits.

Ribwort plantain
Plantago lanceolata

HARVEST TIME
All year-round
FAMILY
Plantaginaceae
COMMON NAME
Lesser plantain

Medicinally, plantain is a powerful little plant, with wind-pollinated white flowers sitting proudly atop long thin stems that seem to dance in the breeze.

As the binomial name *lanceolata* would suggest, the leaves of ribwort plantain are lance shaped, and grow to form an upwards rosette from its base. The short-stemmed leaves have three to five parallel veins or ribs running down the length, which can be separated for cordage making. Compact, oval flower heads are made up of tiny individual flowers with yellow anthers, and can often be seen with a 'halo' of tiny white flowers. Thanks to its natural antihistamine and antiseptic properties, ribwort plantain is a well-known remedy for stings and insect bites. Chewing or rolling the leaves releases the healing juices; alternatively, steep dried leaves in oil and blend with beeswax for a soothing salve that can double up as a drawing ointment. It is a useful plant for smokers or those with bronchitis as it can act as an expectorant, open airways and help to repair damaged lung tissue, while supporting the immune system. The slim leaves make a great substitute for plasters. Plantain tea can be made from fresh or dried leaves to treat allergies. The leaves can also be dried and ground into flour or eaten fresh – they taste like mushroom.

Ribwort plantain thrives in grasslands, fields, park edges, pathways and waste ground from early spring through to early winter. Harvest flower heads in spring and summer; the seeds once they have matured in autumn; the leaves all year-round.

LOOKALIKE: **Greater plantain (*Plantago major*)**

Greater plantain
Plantago major

The larger cousin of ribwort plantain, greater plantain can be differentiated by its wide, rounded leaves and tall flower stalks.

Similar to its cousin, greater plantain boasts many of the same medicinal properties, containing vitamins A, C and K, as well as trace minerals zinc, sodium, calcium, potassium and silica, and also the bitter compounds triterpenes and polysaccharides. The large leaves make for an excellent hot compress, helping to reduce swelling, relieve tired muscles and stop bleeding.

As food, the leaves can be boiled or steamed, though it is best to remove the stringy veins that run down each leaf. The long seed spikes are covered in tiny flowers with purple anthers, which quickly swell into brown seeds rich in proteins, carbohydrates and omega 3 fatty acids. They make a wonderful nutty addition to breads, crackers, cakes, cereals, smoothies, pancakes and anything else that could benefit from a handful of seeds.

These perennials can often be found growing alongside each other in fields, parks, gardens and waste grounds. As with ribwort, harvest flower heads in spring and summer; the seeds once they have matured in autumn; the leaves all year-round.

HARVEST TIME
All year-round
FAMILY
Plantaginaceae
COMMON NAMES
Broadleaf plantain, white man's footprint

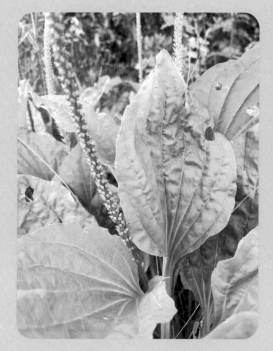

LOOKALIKE: **Ribwort plantain**
(*Plantago lanceolata*)

Wild marjoram
Origanum vulgare

HARVEST TIME
June to Aug
FAMILY
Lamiaceae

Much more than just a sweet, somewhat spiced herb to flavour food, a sprinkling of wild marjoram can also help to aid digestion, accelerate metabolism and promote gut health.

A perennial growing to around 30–60cm (12–24in) tall, wild marjoram has aromatic, oval- or spade-shaped leaves covered in fine hairs. Finely toothed serrated edges appear smooth and, as with most members of the mint family, the leaves are arranged opposite one another on square stems. Blooming in summer through to early autumn, tiny white to pinkish-purple flowers are clustered on flowering stems.

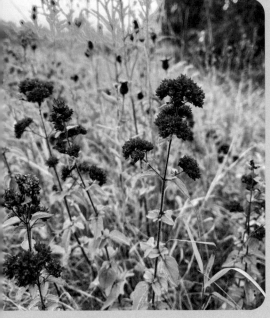

Wild marjoram can help to reduce headaches and anxiety, alleviate symptoms of bruxism (grinding or clenching teeth) and is used to treat sinus problems, reduce inflammation and soothe menstrual cramps. It is antimicrobial and contains iron, as well as vitamins A, E and K.

A classic way to use wild marjoram is fresh on top of pizzas, but a jam or pesto can be made from it too. Make a herbal tea by steeping ¼ tsp dried leaves in a cup of water and add a teaspoon of honey if desired. Fresh herbs can be dried and stored, or preserved in oil, butter or vinegar.

Find wild marjoram on infertile, alkaline soils, or in grassland, hedge banks, woodland edges and scrub land. For best flavour, harvest leaves before the plant comes into flower.

LOOKALIKES:
**Sweet marjoram
(*Origanum
majorana*),
pot marjoram
(*Origanum onites*)**

Chanterelle
Cantharellus cibarius

Chanterelles are a gourmet edible mushroom with a fruity, apricot aroma. When you cut the mushrooms open, the flesh will be white and firm – this is an important feature as the flesh of toxic false chanterelles is the same colour throughout.

Chanterelles are a golden egg-yolk colour; the cap is convex at first, eventually becoming funnel shaped. Mature mushrooms often have wavy, undulating cap margins. There are distinctive wrinkles, or folds, beneath the cap, known as false gills; they should be thick, blunt and decurrent, running down into the short stout stipe. If you're unsure whether you have true or false gills, run your fingers over them and if they easily move back and forth, or crumble, then you have true gills.

These mushrooms are delicious pan-fried and added to pasta sauces. The fruity flavour means they can be used in sweet foods such as marmalades and shortbread, and the firm texture makes them great candidates for pickling and dehydrating.

As a mycorrhizal mushroom, they grow alongside certain species of tree in a symbiotic relationship, most commonly under spruce, pine, beech and birch. A water source and soils with a low pH make for happy chanterelles, so if you find a stream and bilberries in the area too, then you might be on to a good patch.

HARVEST TIME
June to Oct
FAMILY
Cantharellaceae
COMMON NAMES
Girolles, golden chanterelles, golden nuggets
SPORE PRINT
Creamy/ yellowish white

LOOKALIKE: ☠ False chanterelle
(*Hygrophoropsis aurantiaca*)

Fairy ring champignon
Marasmius oreades

HARVEST TIME
Apr to Nov
FAMILY
Marasmiaceae
COMMON NAMES
Resurrection mushroom, mousseron, Scotch bonnet
SPORE PRINT
White

These small mushrooms are known for their whimsical tendency to form fairy rings in grassy areas. The smooth, hygrophanous cap is tan to brown, depending on the weather – when dry they can appear very pale.

The fairy ring's cap is 2–6cm (¾–2¼in) in diameter and convex when young, turning flat with age but usually maintaining its broad umbo. The off-white gills of younger mushrooms turn a dull to creamy pale brown when mature. The flesh is firm and white, the stem slender but tough with no annulus.

Fairy ring champignon have a mildly sweet taste and are one of the best mushrooms for both dehydrating and lactofermenting due to their high levels of trehalose, a glucose that protects cells from drought and high salinity levels. Once rehydrated, these mushrooms can actually go on to sporulate and reproduce!

These mushrooms often form circular or arc-shaped patterns in cut or short, grazed grassy areas – lawns, fields and meadows – from spring throughout summer and often until autumn.

LOOKALIKES:
☠ Fool's funnel
(*Clitocybe rivulosa*),
☠ ivory funnel
(*Clitocybe dealbata*)

Musk mallow

Malva moschata

Musk mallow is a perennial herb with attractive pink or white flowers known for their musky fragrance.

HARVEST TIME
May to Sept
FAMILY
Malvaceae

The open funnel-shaped flowers are 5–7cm (2–2¾in) across, with five pink or white petals, and are arranged in clusters. Lower leaves are heart shaped, with upper leaves having deeply cut palmate lobes.

The high levels of mucilage throughout the plant gives musk mallow its soothing properties and makes it particularly useful for respiratory issues. Crushed leaves can be applied direct to the skin to soothe insect bites and stings. Roots can be boiled into a tea to soothe sore throats and stomach complaints.

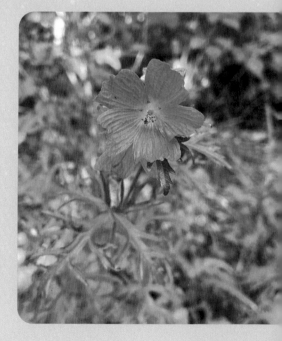

The entire plant is edible and incredibly nutritious, being high in magnesium, potassium and calcium, and containing vitamins A, B and C. Leaves can be eaten raw in salads or, better yet, wilted as a green. Small seeds are fiddly to harvest but lovely sprinkled on baked goods. Flowers are beautiful added to salads, seeming to melt in your mouth, while roots can be used as a soup thickener.

Musk mallow is commonly planted in gardens but can also be found growing wild in meadows, roadsides and disturbed areas, blooming from late spring to early autumn.

LOOKALIKES: **Other mallows (*Malva* spp.)**

Feverfew

Tanacetum parthenium

Feverfew is a medicinal herb with small, daisy-like flowers acclaimed for its long historical use in helping to treat fevers and headaches.

HARVEST TIME
Apr to Sept
FAMILY
Asteraceae
COMMON NAME
Featherfew

This hardy perennial typically grows to 40–80cm (16–31in) tall, with feathery, aromatic fern-like leaves, and umbel-like clusters of small flowers with ivory white petals and a yellow button-like centre.

Feverfew is prescribed by today's herbalists to not only alleviate symptoms of fevers and migraines, but also as a preventative measure. A balm made from the flowers can help sooth inflamed skin, rashes and insect bites. Feverfew has been known to induce menstruation and labour in high doses.

All parts of the plant are edible: the leaves have a fairly bitter flavour but with notes of citrus, and are good chopped and mixed into salads or used to impart an aromatic flavour to foods and beverages; the cute flowers are perfect as a garnish.

Often found in gardens, waste ground, fields, pastures and along roadside verges, from late April through to November, typically flowering between May and September.

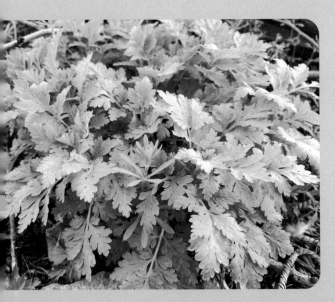

LOOKALIKES: **Chamomile (*Matricaria chamomilla*), oxeye daisy (*Leucanthemum vulgare*)**

Feverfew tincture

A few drops of feverfew tincture a day can help to reduce feelings of melancholy and vertigo, as well as soothe muscle spasms, rheumatism, arthritis and general aches and pains.

Fresh feverfew leaves
and flowers
High-proof alcohol
(i.e. vodka or gin)

1. Fill a clean jar with the leaves and flowers you have harvested.

2. Cover with the alcohol.

3. Leave to infuse for two to four weeks before straining and bottling.

Feverfew tea

A cooled tea can be used as a pain relieving mouth swish for toothache, and has been found effective in the treatment of earache.

Dried or fresh feverfew plant
Boiling water

1. Pour boiling water over the dried or fresh feverfew plant.

2. Steep for 30 minutes.

Caution
As a uterine stimulant, it is not recommended to take feverfew while pregnant. Those on blood-thinning medication should also take caution.

July

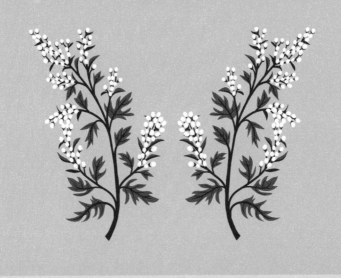

A sun worshipper, I crave the open spaces of fields and meadows during the height of summer – lying on the sun-kissed knoll where wildflowers and quaking grasses stretch overhead creating a natural canopy of colour and delicate whispers in the breeze. Watching vivid beetles wind their way between cornflower stems, and insects of every shape, size and colour clambering over poppies, knapweed, and yarrow in seek of pollen, can almost seem as though you have been transported to another, very distant world.

Frothy meadowsweet fills the air with a honey-sweet scent; white marbled butterflies can be seen flittering around the purple nectar-rich flowers of marjoram, with the small skipper seeming to favour the yellow florets of rough hawkbit.

The encompassing forests not only offer a cooling respite from the midsummer heat but also have now transformed into a bountiful haven of wild sustenance, surpassing the delicate greens of spring. Golden chanterelles, plump boletes and enormous parasol mushrooms are just a few of the fungi to be found in July, with wild strawberries, raspberries and a few early blackberries providing a taste of summer sweetness.

Honesty

Lunaria annua

HARVEST TIME
All year-round
FAMILY
Brassicaceae
COMMON NAMES
Moonwort, penny
flower, two-
pennies-in-a-purse,
money-in-both-
pockets

The honesty plant is a common garden escapee with simple flowers and beautiful pearlescent, disc-shaped seed heads, and has long been used in herbal medicine.

This mainly annual plant can grow to 1m (3ft) high, with stems that are square and hairy. Alternate leaves are large and heart shaped, with a toothed serration. Flowers can be seen in late spring and early summer and are purple, white or a pinkish mix. As with all *Brassicas*, the flowers are simple, with four petals, and located on terminal racemes. These flowers are followed by the distinctive seed pods that start off as green discs before transforming into translucent ivory windows that remain on the plant, even after the paper sheaf holding the seeds in place falls off.

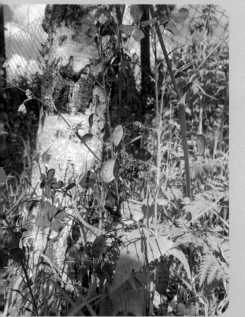

Medicinally, honesty is used to treat coughs, sore throats and bronchitis, as well as to help alleviate menstrual cramps and support reproductive health. As a *Brassica*, the plant has a spicy kick; the young leaves and green developing seed pods can be eaten raw or cooked, and the seeds can be mixed with cider vinegar and honey for a mustard substitute. The flowers can be used as a spicy garnish to meals, and to create a natural dye that can range from pale purple to deep blue depending on the mordant used.

Harvest honesty all year-round: the leaves in spring; flowers in summer; seeds in autumn; and roots in winter.

LOOKALIKES: **Other *Brassicas* before flowering**

Mugwort
Artemisia vulgaris

A large plant with a distinctive sage-like aroma, mugwort has long been considered a magical herb, used as a sedative and to promote vivid dreaming.

HARVEST TIME
All year-round
FAMILY
Asteraceae
COMMON NAMES
Midge wort,
maiden's wort,
sailor's tobacco,
bollan bane

Reaching up to 1.5m (5ft), mugwort has a green to reddish-purple grooved stem, which turns reddish-brown and woody with age. Pinnate leaves are alternate and are more deeply lobed at the top of the plant, with undersides covered with soft silver hairs, while upper leaf surfaces are smooth or slightly hairy. Tiny white flowers are inconspicuous on short stalks, and occur on tall, bellowing, spiked clusters at the top of the plant.

Mugwort is a helpful plant for menstruation, relaxing the uterus, relieving cramps and regulating the menstrual cycle. It also has the ability to delay menstruation and to induce abortions – so should not be taken during pregnancy. It can be made into a salve or compress to help arthritis and reduce itchiness from raised scars. Mugwort can be dried for medicinal teas and tinctures to help ease digestive complaints and regulate blood pressure.

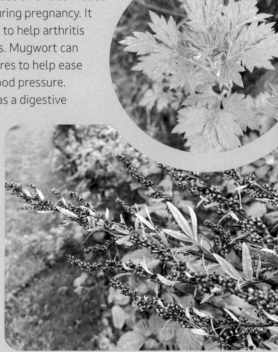

As a wild food, it is often served as a digestive aid alongside fatty foods, and is used to flavour everything from vegetables, fish and meats, to soups, salads and desserts.

Harvest leaves in summer before the plant goes into flower; flowers in late summer; and roots in autumn or winter.

LOOKALIKES:
☠ Wolfsbane (*Aconitum napellus*), wormwood (*Artemisia absinthium*)

Wild cherry
Prunus avium

This deciduous tree bears beautiful white, almond-scented blossom each spring and small edible fruits that are a favourite of birds and foragers alike.

HARVEST TIME
Mar to Aug
FAMILY
Rosaceae
COMMON NAMES
Sweet cherry,
gean, bird cherry

The straight trunk is covered in a smooth, grey or reddish-brown bark with narrow horizontal lines, lenticels, etched into its bark. These act as pores, helping gases to flow through. The glossy green leaves are oval to elliptical, with sharply toothed serrated edges, pointed tips, veins and two red glands at the top of the petiole. Flowers are white with five petals, usually hanging in clusters of between two and six. The fleshy stone fruits are smaller than cultivated cherries, are dark red in colour and have a sweet to slightly sour taste.

Cherries are high in antioxidants and protect and heal the cells in our body, as well as inhibit oxidation and remove toxins. They contain essential fatty acids and promote brain and vision function, as well as relieving arthritis and hypertension, while regulating both the immune and central nervous systems. Cherries are also anti-inflammatory and promote the formation of collagen, reducing redness and improving skin elasticity. Cherry fruits and their leaves contain melatonin, which promotes sleep, making a great bedtime tea. Use an infusion of stalks to treat chest complaints.

Infuse wild cherries into liqueurs, and make the blossom into a syrup for drinks and desserts, or skin-soothing tonics, toners and sugar scrubs. Boil cherry pits with sugar and water into a syrup, or reduce further with red wine for an almond-flavoured glaze.

Find cherry trees in parks, gardens, old woodlands, along hedgerows and lining streets. All *Prunus* are edible, though some are too tart to eat the berries raw. Harvest flowers in spring, but leave plenty to turn into fruits in early summer.

LOOKALIKES:
Sour cherry
(*Prunus cerasus*),
Cherry plum
(*Prunus cerasifera*),
other ornamental
cherries and
hybrids

Black mustard

Brassica nigra

If you love a kick to your salad, then black mustard is one to look out for. Mustard plants release a chemical compound when damaged, giving the characteristic pungent flavour.

HARVEST TIME
Mar to Nov
FAMILY
Brassicaceae
COMMON NAME
Wild mustard

Growing up to 2m (6ft), for most of the year the black mustard plant is much smaller. From April, clusters of yellow cruciform flowers grow near to and at the ends of thin branching stems, developing into green, elongated, two-chambered seed pods containing small, rounded black seeds. Basal leaves are large and pinnately lobed, with a larger terminal lobe and an irregularly serrated margin; upper leaves are smaller and unlobed; linear leaves sit beneath the flowering stems.

Black mustard is a source of trace elements and vitamins A, B1, B2 and C. The flowering tops are one of the most nutritious parts of the plant and can be cooked like sprouting broccoli. The flowers also make a colourful garnish. The underside of mature leaves are coated in stiff white hairs so are best harvested young for use in salads or as a herb. Larger leaves can be cooked, though do become bitter. Seeds are easiest to gather when the pods are still green: pop them in a paper bag and let them dry outside for a week or so before storing in a spice jar. They can be ground into powder to season food or flavour wine, mixed with oil and vinegar to make mustard sauce, or added to pickles and ferments.

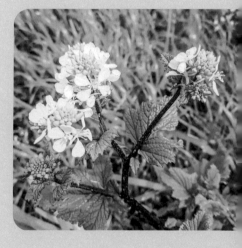

Harvest when leaves first appear in early spring, typically March; flowers can be harvested in early summer; seeds from early autumn until November. Find black mustard in fields, roadsides or wasteland – it thrives in disturbed areas.

LOOKALIKE:
**Field mustard
(*Brassica rapa*)**

Water lily
Nymphaea spp.

Water lilies are aquatic plants that thrive in water and damp, marshy soil. Not only are the flowers edible, but they are also used as a calming sedative.

HARVEST TIME
Mar to Sept
FAMILY
Nymphaeaceaee

Firmly anchored by roots and rhizomes in the muddy substrate, these plants send stems reaching to 3m (10ft). Above the water's surface emerge large round leaves that feature a waxy, water-repellent coating and display a distinct V-shaped notch at the point where the petiole attaches. Highly fragrant flowers are white, pink or yellow depending on species.

Targeting the nervous system, water lily flowers have a relaxing and sedative effect, reputedly reducing the sex drive and making them a useful plant for those who suffer with insomnia or anxiety.

The whole plant can be eaten: flowers are edible raw and can be used in salads or rice rolls; unopened buds can be boiled or pickled; stems can be eaten like asparagus; seeds can be ground for use in baking or as a coffee substitute; young shoots can be chopped and added to soups, stews and stir fries, with the larger ones being useful for cooking and/or wrapping food – and they make handy plates for riverside picnics too.

Cut young leaves and flower buds in spring and early summer. Fruits and seeds can be collected in late summer and early autumn, and tubers are best harvested before the plant comes into flower.

Caution
Water lilies affect the nervous system, so small amounts are advised.

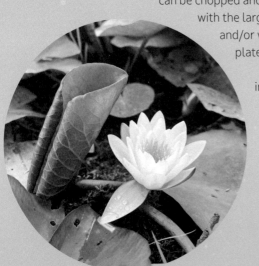

Wild raspberry
Rubus idaeus

The five-petalled white flowers of the raspberry plant transform into the classic bobbly, aggregate red summer fruit we all know and love, and it's not uncommon to pick a few stray berries until first frosts.

A perennial evergreen shrub, the stems take the form of upright or slightly arching canes bearing small thorns or prickles. Canes can grow up to 1.5m (5ft). Leaves are pinnate, with leaflets usually ovate to lanceolate, with a serrated edge and bright green, but paler on the underside.

Raspberry leaf has a long tradition of use with late-term pregnancy that continues to this day, helping to strengthen the muscles of the womb, aiding delivery and increasing the production of breast milk. Raspberry leaves are rich in vitamins, minerals and antioxidants, and are especially high in iron, manganese and chlorogenic acid.

Harvest new shoots and leaves in spring while young and tender; berries ripen from early summer until autumn.

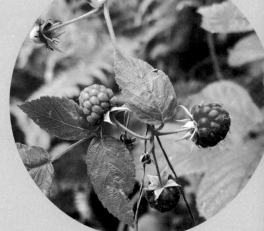

HARVEST TIME
May to July
FAMILY
Rosaceae
COMMON NAME
Hindberry
(Scotland)

Raspberry leaf tea
- *1 tbsp dried leaves per cup of warm water*

Cover and steep for 5–10 minutes. If you wish to add a sweetener, then a little organic honey would preserve the beneficial herbal compounds of the raspberry leaf.

LOOKALIKE:
Blackberry
(*Rubus fruticosus*)

Elderflower & raspberry leaf iced tea

Raspberry leaf tea has the familiar comfort of black tea, but the elderflower gives this thirst-quenching summer's drink a gentle, floral flavour.

This refreshing drink is perfect for sun-soaked days in the garden, or, better yet, poured into an insulated bottle full of ice and taken with you on those balmy evening woodland walks.

Elderflower syrup:
150g (5oz) sugar
350ml (12fl oz) water
3 large sprays of fresh
  elderflowers
Sprig of lemon balm

Iced tea:
12 to 15 young, fresh
  raspberry leaves
1 litre (2 pints) water
Ice cubes
100ml (3fl oz)
  elderflower syrup
500ml (1 pint) cooled tea

To make the elderflower syrup:

1. Heat the sugar and water until all of the sugar has dissolved.

2. Remove elderflowers from stems with a fork, add to the syrup with the lemon balm and leave to infuse in the fridge for 12–48 hours.

To make the iced tea:

1. Steep raspberry leaves in boiling water and leave to cool.

2. Fill a pitcher with plenty of ice.

3. Add 100ml (3fl oz) elderflower syrup and 500ml (1 pint) cooled tea, and stir.

4. Garnish with lemon slices, cucumber strips or flower springs and enjoy in the sunshine!

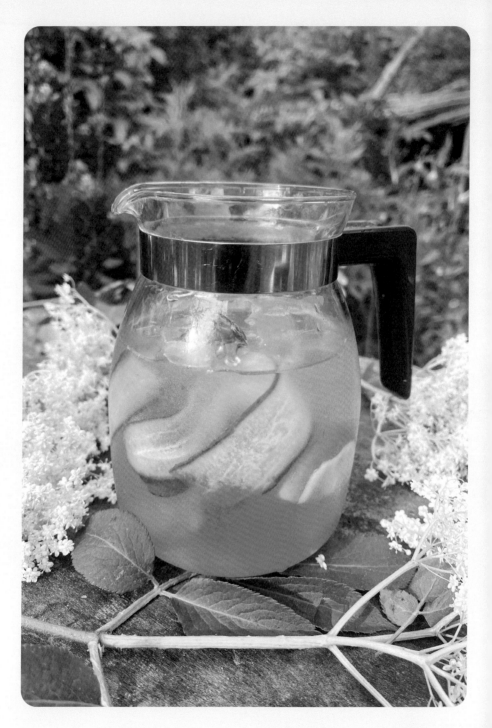

Sweet cicely
Myrrhis odorata

HARVEST TIME
All year-round
FAMILY **Apiaceae**
COMMON NAMES
**Sweet chervil, wild
myrrh, sweet fern,
sweet hemlock**

All parts of this plant have a strong aniseed scent, so a simple crush-and-smell will tell you if you have sweet cicely or a potentially toxic lookalike (see below).

Sweet cicely is a tall plant reaching up to 1m (3ft), with bright green, pinnate, fern-like leaves covered in tiny hairs, giving them a soft velvety feel. Flowers are small, have five petals and are arranged in umbels that form larger, compound umbels.

Sweet cicely has a long and hollow tap root which can be dried and made into a tea to improve the appetite, purify the blood and treat the formation of intestinal gas. The root can also be infused into oil and made into an ointment to help heal wounds and promote healing.

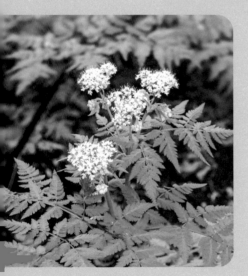

The sweet and juicy stems contain the flavonoid anethole, which is 13 times sweeter than sugar, making this a plant that lends itself well to desserts. Leaves can be infused into milk, cream or custard, or chopped and eaten fresh in salads. Seeds have a strong liquorice flavour and are great freshly infused into spirits, dried and crumbled on desserts, or used as a spice, similar to fennel seed.

A common perennial, you can find sweet cicely growing among hedgerows, in park and field edges, in damp meadows, on roadsides and as a garden escapee. Harvest leaves and roots all year-round, flowers from May to July and seeds in August.

LOOKALIKES:
☠ Poison hemlock (*Conium maculatum*), cow parsley (*Anthriscus sylvestris*), wild fennel (*Foeniculum vulgare*)

Wild fennel

Foeniculum vulgare

Wild fennel is a tall and aromatic biennial herb smelling strongly of liquorice, with delicately feathery leaves and umbrella-like clusters of yellow flowers.

HARVEST TIME
Apr to Oct
FAMILY
Apiaceae
COMMON NAME
Sweet fennel

An upright branching perennial reaching 2m (6½ft) in height, the leaves of wild fennel appear from April. The deeply divided grey-green leaves have a lacy appearance, and leaf stems are enveloped in a pale sheath at the base. Tall spikes of smooth, finely furrowed stems carry loose umbels of vibrant yellow clusters that bloom from July through to October and develop into green, elongated ovoid seed pods.

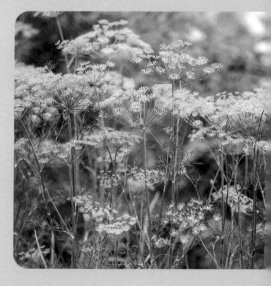

The entire plant is edible and has a sweet but unmistakable aniseed aroma, making wild fennel one of the few members of the Apiaceae family that's easy to identify. Wild fennel doesn't produce a bulb, but you can get the same flavour from the young shoots, leaves, seeds, flowers and even the pollen, if you feel up to the finnicky challenge of collecting it! However, it is the seeds that are used for medicine, containing an essential oil with anethole and fenchone as the main constituents, alongside flavonoids and coumarins. Herbal teas made with fennel seed are often prescribed for upper respiratory diseases and digestive tract issues, but they can also be cooled and used as an eyewash for conjunctivitis and styes. Fennel seed also makes for an awesome post-meal digestive aid.

Wild fennel thrives in wasteland, disturbed areas, hedgerows and field edges, and alongside riverbanks and railway tracks.

Marsh woundwort
Stachys palustris

Don't let the smell of marsh woundwort put you off – it is a delightful little edible plant with valuable food and medicine offerings from spring until winter.

HARVEST TIME
Year-round
FAMILY
Lamiaceae
COMMON NAMES
Marsh hedge
nettle, clown
woundwort

A fairly low-growing plant rarely reaching more than 1m (40in), the spike-like clusters of marsh woundwort's flowers whorl around the hairy, square stem. Lilac-coloured flowers are tubular and hooded, with the upper lip covered in short, fine hairs, and three lower lobes. Velvety green leaves are oblong to lanceolate, bluntly serrated and arranged in opposing pairs.

March woundwort is an antihistamine, antiseptic, anti-inflammatory and also an excellent styptic: crushed leaves can be applied topically as a poultice to stem bleeding and heal wounds. A herbal tea made from the leaves and flowers can be taken both internally and externally for cramp relief, joint pain and mild sedative effects.

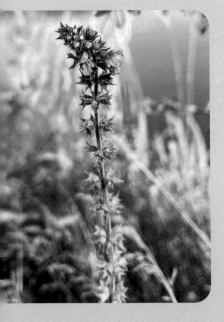

Leaves and flowering tops can be lightly cooked. The tubers are like an elongated version of Chinese artichokes and can be eaten in much the same way – raw, boiled, roasted, pan fried or dried into a baking flour. They have a nutty flavour and cooking removes any bitterness. Flowers and seeds are also edible and make a nutritious salad topping.

With new shoots appearing in early spring and flowers in July and August, harvest marsh woundwort as it comes into flower in July; the tubers in autumn or winter. Found in damp meadows, riverbanks, ditches, marshes and along water edges.

LOOKALIKE: **Hedge woundwort**
(*Stachys sylvatica*)

Common chicory
Cichorium intybus

Chicory is the parent plant from which lots of our cultivated varieties are bred, giving its trademark bitterness to leafy greens such as radicchio and endive.

HARVEST TIME
Mar to Nov
FAMILY
Asteraceae
COMMON NAMES
Wild chicory,
blue daisy,
blue dandelion,
coffee weed

Chicory is a branching herbaceous plant blooming between June and October with bright blue flowers that have raggedly notched petals, which can occasionally be white. Leaves are variable: basal leaves are often deeply lobed and irregularly toothed; upper leaves are usually lanceolate and can be either toothed or entire and grow alternately up a tough, grooved stem.

This bitter leaf is high in fibre and inulin, packed full of gut-friendly prebiotics and exceptionally rich in vitamin A, potassium and folic acid. Leaves can be made into a poultice for swelling and inflammation. Young leaves can be added raw to salads or sandwiches; when the plant comes into flower, the more palatable option would be to wilt leaves in butter. Chicory root can be roasted and ground as a caffeine-free coffee, and indeed became a substitute for instant coffee during World War II, giving it the common name of coffee weed. The roasted roots can also be infused into milk or cream to impart an earthy, caramel-like flavour. A blue dye can be extracted from the leaves, an orange dye from the roots.

Harvest leaves in spring, flowers in summer and roots in autumn. Found in woodland edges, waste ground, roadside verges, alleyways and disturbed areas, chicory loves to grow in compacted soil, so be prepared to dig!

LOOKALIKE: **Dandelion (*Taraxacum*, before flowering)**

Devil's bit scabious

Succisa pratensis

This purple-blue wildflower was traditionally used to treat scabies, but now its uses extend to treating respiratory ailments.

HARVEST TIME
Mar to Sept
FAMILY
Caprifoliaceae
COMMON NAMES
Blue button,
devil's pincushion

This slow-growing perennial reaches 60–90cm (2–3ft) in height. Heads of tiny, tubular flowers are arranged in dense pompom-like clusters with prominent anthers. Flower heads sit at the top of thin stems, blooming from July to early November, with flowers eventually forming spiky seed heads in late autumn into winter. Basal leaves are elliptical and typically unserrated, while upper leaves are serrated and pinnate.

Scabious were traditionally used to treat scabies, however the famed 17th-century London herbalist Nicholas Culpeper (1616–54) prescribed the plant as an antidote for snake venom by boiling the roots; a concoction that also proved to be helpful in the treatment of coughs, sore throats and respiratory issues. Young leaves and shoots can be eaten raw or added to salads, flower buds can be pickled like capers and opened flowers make a pretty salad topper.

Found in meadows, damp grassland and woodland, fields, pastures and moorland. Look out for the marsh fritillary butterfly and the narrow-bordered bee hawk-moth, which dine on it.

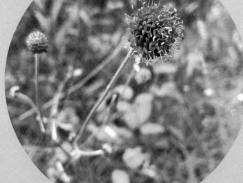

LOOKALIKES:
Macedonian scabious (*Knautia macedonica*)
and other *Scabious* spp.

Chicken of the woods
Laetiporus sulphureus

One of the most well-known mushrooms due to its bright colour, large, cartoon-like appearance and uncanny texture of chicken.

Velvet-textured caps are orange or sulphur-yellow, reminiscent of candy corn, with white to pale yellow pores on the underside. Growing to around 50cm (20in) in diameter, in fan-shaped tiers or overlapping brackets with an undulating margin, most commonly on oak, but also found on beech, sweet chestnut, cherry and willow.

As the name would imply, chicken of the woods has a firm, fibrous and meaty texture that can be marinated for use as a chicken substitute. Harvest young specimens, as older mushrooms become tough and leathery. This mushroom is rich in vitamin C and potassium, and a healthy amount of carbohydrates, protein, fibre and fats, making it a great meat substitute. Try dipping in egg wash and a breadcrumb batter for a plant-based schnitzel.

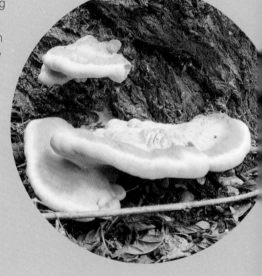

HARVEST TIME
May to Nov
FAMILY
Fomitopsidaceae
COMMON NAME
Sulphur polypore
SPORE PRINT
White

Caution
• *It is not recommended to harvest chicken of the woods from the toxic common yew tree as, although unlikely, there may be a risk of deadly toxin transfer.*

• *Around 1 in 10 people suffer gastrointestinal upset after ingesting chicken of the woods. As with all wild food, try a small amount and wait 24 hours before cooking any for dinner.*

LOOKALIKES: **Blackening polypore (Meripilus giganteus)**, **hen of the woods (Grifola frondosa)**

Sneezewort

Achillea ptarmica

If yarrow and feverfew had a child, it would be the perennial wildflower, sneezewort, recognized by its strong scent when crushed, branching habit and the loose clusters of daisy-like flower heads.

Notched, white petals surround a pincushion-like central disc of tubular florets. Greyish-green leaves are slender and lanceolate, with sharply serrated margins, and grow in an alternate arrangement on downy stems.

Sneezewort has a herbal, almost pepper-like flavour; the roots can be dried, ground and prepared into a tea to help reduce joint pain and arthritis. The leaves can be cooked or eaten raw, though fresh ones do create a numbing, tingling effect, which can be used to provide pain relief to toothache or ulcers. Leaves can also be crushed and applied directly to the skin as both an insect repellent and anti-inflammatory poultice, and fresh leaves and flowers can be added to baths for a herbal soak.

Harvest flowers from June to September, and roots once the plant has finished blooming. Found in damp meadows, pastures, field edges and waste grounds.

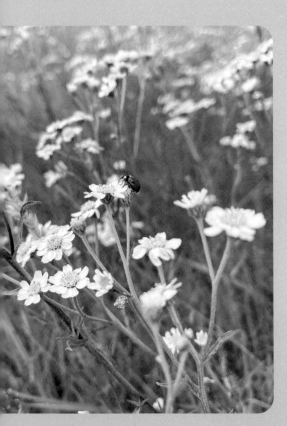

LOOKALIKES:
Feverfew (*Tanacetum parthenium*),
yarrow (*Achillea millefolium*)

Evening primrose
Oenothera biennis

Evening primrose is a common and hardy medicinal wildflower known for its showy yellow flowers that bloom in the evening. The entire plant is edible and the seeds are particularly medicinally beneficial.

HARVEST TIME
All year-round
FAMILY
Onagraceae
COMMON NAMES
Evening star, sun
drop, king's
cure-all

In the first year, this biennial produces a rosette of leaves; and in the second year, it sends up tall flowering stems. Alternate leaves are elliptical to lanceolate, with a white or pink midrib, short petiole and slightly toothed or wavy margin. Fairly large sessile flowers have four bright yellow petals with an x-shaped stigma, flowering from late spring to late summer. After flowering, cylindrical seed capsules develop. These hairy, erect capsules split open to release the seeds.

The seeds are small but are known for their oil content, which is a rich source of gamma-linolenic acid, an essential fatty acid found in breast milk believed to have anti-inflammatory properties helping to treat skin issues, premenstrual pain, asthma, eczema and arthritis. A tea can be made from the flowers and leaves to help aid dietary issues, while a hot poultice made from the root can be applied externally to bruises and boils.

Young leaves can be lightly cooked or added fresh to salads. The taproot can be harvested and cooked once the plant has finished flowering: wash it, peel off the outer layer and roast or boil – they have a starchy, slightly sweet taste and contain protein and dietary fibre. Seeds can be consumed raw, toasted or ground into a powder.

Gather tender leaves in spring before the plant starts flowering. Can be found in waste ground, roadsides, meadows, dry soil and open ground.

August

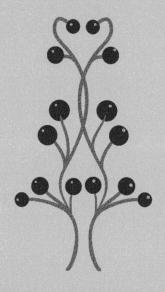

The sun is high, the days are long and winter seems a million miles away. Heather blankets the moorlands as far as the eye can see, shimmering in shades of lavender and mauve. Among the purple, crowberries, cowberries and bilberries can all be spotted ripening, sheep sorrel and wild thyme are nestled between the rocks, while down in the valleys the autumn fungi are starting to knock at the door.

Mugwort and wormwood are in flower along field edges, giant puffballs litter the grass like lost footballs, baubles of cherry plums decorate the trees, red hawthorn berries festoon the hedgerows, and the silvery threads of old man's beard entwine gracefully around the wild rose bushes, as their hips begin to fatten.

Listen closely and you might notice the sound of distant fireworks as the ripe seed pods of chickweed, stitchwort and gorse explode under the intensity of the summer sun. August is a superb time for collecting dry seed heads to create a wildflower garden the following year, sprinkled around the surrounding meadows to help ensure next year's harvest, or even sprouted at home – try seeds such as black mustard, fat hen and curly dock for nutrient-dense micro-greens.

Crowberry
Empetrum nigrum

HARVEST TIME
June to Mar
FAMILY
Ericaceae
COMMON NAMES
Crawberry,
crawcrooks,
mossberry

Though bitter in taste, crowberries are high in antioxidants, fibre, folate and vitamins C and K, so they are definitely worth collecting if you stumble across a good patch.

A creeping, matted, evergreen shrub, crowberry has short, stubby, light green leaves, which are fleshy and needle-like, with a trailing growth habit. The leaves are deeply grooved beneath with edges that roll under. Small pinkish-purple flowers with five petals are borne into the axil of the leaves. Crowberry has small, shiny black berries when ripe.

Containing some of the highest levels of antioxidants of all the wild berries, crowberries are a valuable source of anthocyanins and polyphenols, which help to protect the body from disease and oxidative stress. The high concentration of anthocyanin pigment also makes crowberries an awesome natural food dye. Alternatively, mix into granola or with other berries, or make into jams, jellies, sauces and syrups.

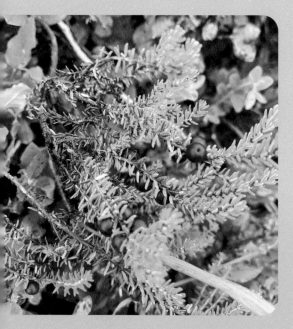

High in tannins, this is a berry that sweetens when eaten after the first frosts; luckily, berries often hang around well into the depths of winter. Berries that do overwinter can be collected in the spring.

LOOKALIKE: **Bilberry**
(*Vaccinium myrtillus*)

Himalayan balsam
Impatiens glandulifera

As a potentially invasive plant, care must be taken when harvesting Himalayan balsam, and seeds are best carried home in a sealed container to prevent accidental spreading of the plant.

HARVEST TIME
June to Oct
FAMILY
Balsaminaceae
COMMON NAMES
Indian balsam, jumping Jack, policeman's helmet, kiss-me-on-the-mountain, jewelweed

This fast-growing, fast-spreading annual plant can tower above head-height, with smooth, hollow, hexagonal stems (which can be used as drinking straws). Nodding clusters of magenta, and occasionally white or purple, flowers form the shape of an old-fashioned policeman's helmet, which gives them one of their common names. The flowers are followed by seed pods which, when ripe, audibly explode upon the slightest touch and are fun to watch on a windy day! The lanceolate leaves are green with sharply toothed red edges.

The leaves are cooling in nature and can be used as a poultice to treat sunburn and tired muscles. Flowers can be used to make a magical syrup: when the syrup is added to another acidic liquid, such as lemonade or tonic, its colour changes from a pale to vibrant pink. Seeds are light when young, turning black when mature; they can be eaten at any stage and have a nutty taste. Add fresh or dry seeds to curries, make crunchy deep-fried pods as a side, or pickle and preserve.

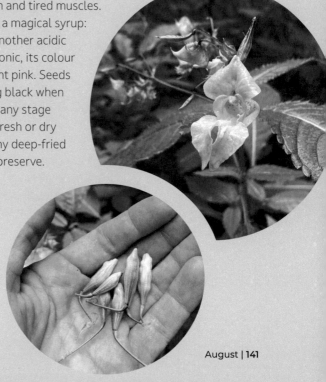

LOOKALIKE:
Rosebay willow-herb
(*Epilobium angustifolium*)

Bilberry
Vaccinium myrtillus

A tiny but more flavoursome version of the imported blueberries we see on the supermarket shelves – not only is the taste more intense, but bilberries also have around four times the antioxidant power.

HARVEST TIME
June to Oct
FAMILY
Ericaceae
COMMON NAMES
Blaeberry, whortleberry, windberry, myrtle berry, whimberry

A low-growing shrub rarely reaching hip height, bright green leaves grow on short stalks, are oval shaped with a pointed tip, and are edged with a tiny-toothed serration. They turn a beautiful deep orange-red before shedding for winter. Small, pink, ballerina-shaped flowers droop from the plants in spring.

The antioxidant power of bilberries comes from their high levels of anthocyanins, making them helpful for cognitive health and protecting against cancer and heart disease. They are also a great source of vitamin C, manganese and fibre, helping to lower cholesterol and regulate blood sugar levels.

The leaves can be used to flavour smoked foods, or fermented and made into tea. The flowers make a pretty garnish, or leave them on the shrub to transform into plump, squishy, deep blue/black berries with a white bloom and red flesh that stains hands and clothes. The dye can be used as a natural food colouring, and to dye fabrics a royal purple.

Find bilberries in moorland, heathland, up on high ground and in acidic woodland. Fruits start ripening in early summer, with a glut in August, and often found until October. For speedy harvesting, brush bushes with a fork or pick comb, with a container beneath.

LOOKALIKE: **Cowberry**
(*Vaccinium vitis-idaea*)

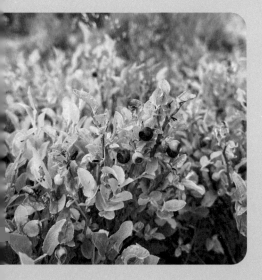

Blackberry

Rubus fruticosus

Depending on location, growing conditions and subspecies, blackberries can taste vastly different from bush to bush, with flavour ranging from sweet to tart to bitter.

HARVEST TIME
Mar to Oct
FAMILY
Rosaceae
COMMON NAMES
Bramble, European blackberry

Blackberries grow on either a vine or shrub with trailing or arching stems that are covered in sharp thorns. Leaves are alternate trifoliate, with three, five, seven or nine deeply serrated leaflets. Pink or white flowers emerge in late spring, going on to form dense green clusters that later ripen to red, then glossy, plump black berries.

Aside from its berries, blackberry offers other delights. Fresh leaves and young stems have a mild nutty flavour. Drying the leaves intensifies the flavour and when steeped in hot water they make a delicious tea that stimulates the appetite, improves blood circulation, acts as a mouthwash and helps to relieve hangovers. Bramble stems can be stripped of their thorns and weaved into a basket, and cordage can be made by bashing the stems to extract the fibres within.

Blackberries produce fruit and seeds without fertilization, a form of reproduction known as apomixis. As a result, some species remain extremely localized. One of the most fun things about foraging blackberries is getting to know which bushes work best for certain dishes. It's said you shouldn't pick them after 19th September, as the devil (in fact, the flesh fly) spits on them (regurgitates) and they become cursed (rot faster). Harvest new shoots and leaves in spring.

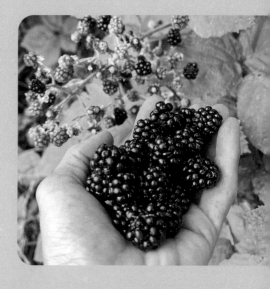

LOOKALIKE:

Wild raspberry (*Rubus idaeus*)

Cherry plum
Prunus cerasifera

HARVEST TIME
June to Sept
FAMILY
Rosaceae
COMMON NAME
Myrobalan plum

With its pretty, almond-scented white blossom, the cherry plum brings the gleeful anticipation of spring, as well as opportunities for reaping its medicinal benefits and delicious fruit.

A deciduous, broadleaf tree reaching heights of 8m (26ft), the cherry plum has dark grey bark, which develops cracks and scars with age. The white flowers have five petals and emerge before the leaves, which are green, glossy and oval shaped with deep, curved veins, a toothed serration and fine hairs on the underside.

A green dye can be extracted from the leaves, while the blossom can be infused into milk for desserts, candied for decoration or steeped into tea to reap the medicinal benefits (it is said to aid with stress, relieve anxiety and halt irrational thoughts or fear of losing control). The round fruits are red, yellow or plum-coloured, are sweet and tasty eaten fresh, and just as delicious when made into jams, chutneys, compotes, wines and syrups.

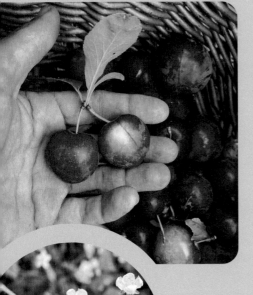

Depending on the variety, fruits ripen from late June until early September. And depending on how sheltered the growing conditions are, and how hungry the local wildlife is, fruits can be found still hanging on the trees until mid-autumn. The cherry plum is a popular ornamental street tree often planted in parks and gardens, and you can also find it growing semi-wild as a shrub or tree in old orchards and woodlands.

LOOKALIKES: Blackthorn (*Prunus spinosa*), black cherry plum (*Prunus cerasifera* 'Nigra')

Field mushroom
Agaricus campestris

Field mushrooms are the most commonly eaten fungi in the UK, and are closely related to the cultivated supermarket button and portobello varieties, *Agaricus bisporous*.

The smooth, sometimes slightly scaly, white to off-white cap starts life looking much like a golf ball lost in the grass, before opening up and flattening out, growing to around 4–10cm (1½–4in) or more in diameter. The somewhat fibrous skin of the cap hangs below the margin slightly, a helpful distinguishing feature. Beneath the cap of young mushrooms you will sometimes find the partial veil still attached, before it comes away to leave behind a small, transient skirt on the stipe, which is 4–8cm (1½–3in) tall. Free, deep pink gills are very crowded, and turn a brown colour when mature.

HARVEST TIME
Apr to Nov
FAMILY
Agaricaceae
COMMON NAME
Meadow mushroom
SPORE PRINT
Deep brown

Field mushrooms can be helpful in treating high cholesterol, type 2 diabetes, bloodstream disorders and osteoporosis. The inside flesh has a pleasant mushroomy aroma, is firm and white, and blushes a pale pink when damaged. The large, firm caps are perfect for stuffing and roasting, filling pies or slicing up and frying in butter for mushrooms on toast.

Field caps can be harvested at any size. Find them growing in chemical-free fields, meadows, lawns, roadside verges, parks and golf courses, and often in fairy rings.

LOOKALIKES **Horse mushroom (*Agaricus arvensis*),**
☠ **yellow stainer (*Agaricus xanthodermus*),**
☠ **destroying angel (*Amanita virosa*)**

Staghorn sumac
Rhus typhina

HARVEST TIME
June to Feb
FAMILY
Anacardiaceae
COMMON NAME
Velvet sumac

Distinctive, dense, dark red bunches of fuzzy berries stand proud on tree branches like candelabras. While the young shoots can be eaten raw, it's the berries that are most widely used, for their delicious, sharp flavour.

The leaves of staghorn sumac are pinnately compound, made up of multiple leaflets with a coarsely toothed edge, in an opposite or slightly alternate arrangement. The upper leaf surface is deep green with a duller green underside. Young branches are covered in fine hairs that resemble the velvet on stag antlers, and the tree puts on a display of vivid crimson hues come autumn.

Staghorn sumac is high in vitamin C and contains dietary fibre, healthy fats and antioxidants. It can be used wherever astringency is needed. Make a sharp, floral tea by steeping the flowers in hot water; cool this to use as a mouthwash to relieve sore gums, or as a face toner to reduce inflammation. The berries are usually dried, crushed and added as a spice or to flavour drinks. Often used as a part of a marinade, sumac contains an enzyme that helps to break down and tenderize meat, while powdered sumac berries make colourful, tangy sugars and salts with a hint of smokiness. Hot water releases the bitter alkaloids present in sumac berries, so a cold-water infusion is best to preserve flavour.

Sumac is commonly planted in parks and gardens where it can sometimes escape into neighbouring fields and woodland edges. Harvest after a few dry days, as it can lose its flavour after heavy rain. Seed pods ripen in summer but remain on the tree throughout winter and can be harvested at any time, as long as they are not too damaged by weather or insects.

Fat hen

Chenopodium album

Fat hen is a common wasteland edible with a mild flavour similar to spinach, to which it is related and used in much the same way.

Typically reaching around 1m (3ft) in height with an upright, branching habit, fat hen sports blue-green, diamond-shaped alternate leaves that have a white, powdery coating on the underside, which is easily rubbed off. The inconspicuous white-green flowers appear in clusters from late summer through autumn.

A topical juice made from the crushed fleshy stems of fat hen can be used to treat sunburn; the crushed roots can be mixed with water and used as a mild soap alternative. The leaves are rich in nutrients and can be used in salads or cooked dishes that call for *Brassica* leaves.

Fat hen contains more iron, protein, calcium, phosphorus and vitamins A, B1, B2 and C than its spinach cousin, so it is well worth taking it back to the kitchen. Eat it alongside beans to act as a carminative. Flowers can be cooked similarly to sprouting broccoli, while seeds can be dried and used as a quinoa substitute.

Fat hen is often found in fields, alongside woodland paths and in disturbed areas, and loves to pop up on any bare soil in gardens. It first appears in February, providing food right up until the winter frosts.

HARVEST TIME
Feb to Oct
FAMILY
Amaranthaceae
COMMON NAMES
Lamb's quarters, wild spinach, goosefoot

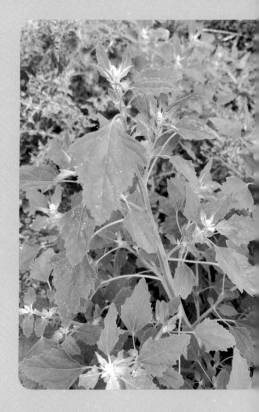

Common puffball
Lycoperdon perlatum

The inside flesh of the puffball is white and spongy like a marshmallow when young, and it is then that these fungi should be harvested. Discard any that are yellow or brown inside, as these will have started to sporulate and will be inedible.

HARVEST TIME
Aug to Dec
FAMILY
Agaricaceae
COMMON NAMES
Warted puffball, jewelled puffball, gem-studded puffball, wolf farts
SPORE PRINT
Olive to dark brown

The warts on the fruit body start off the same colour as the mushroom, then turn yellow to a clay-brown colour, before falling off and leaving a mottling to the surface. As the mushroom gets ready to release its spores, it will develop a darker area in the centre, where a pore hole will appear. When rain hits the mushroom, or it is knocked by a passing paw or foot, billions of spores 'puff' out like little clouds of smoke. The bottom of the mushroom is tapered and often still has the mycelial cords where it was attached to the earth.

The common puffball is recognized for its spores' potential as antimicrobial, antibacterial and antifungal agents. These properties suggest a broader application in combating various illnesses, including E. coli and salmonella. Find puffballs in deciduous and coniferous woodlands, in parks and alongside verges, from late summer through to early winter. They are known to be bioaccumulators (collect pollutants such as pesticides), so shouldn't be harvested near busy roads. Use promptly after harvesting.

LOOKALIKES: **Other** *Lycoperdon*, stinkhorn (*Phallus impudicus*) eggs, ☠ common earthball (*Scleroderma citrinum*)

Caution
Take care when harvesting puffballs as they can be mistaken for Amanita *mushrooms in their egg stage, some of which are poisonous (see page 18). Always cut the mushroom open and check the insides to make sure the flesh is pure white and spongey, with no sign of a hard skin and no other mushroom within.*

Penny bun
Boletus edulis

Seemingly elusive, penny buns are considered one of the tastiest wild mushrooms in the world. They have a viscid-when-wet cap that resembles a freshly baked bread bun, sometimes with a noteably paler cap edge.

Boletes are a genus of mushroom that all (well, mostly) bear a cushion of pores beneath the cap, rather than the classic gills you would usually expect to find. White pores turn cream then yellow with age, and the chunky, bulbous white stipe can be pale brown towards the top and covered in a white netting called reticulation, which is more prominent towards the top of the stipe.

These mushrooms have a umami, earthy flavour and make for an intense seasoning when dried and turned into a powder for use when cooking. Blitzing the powder up with sea salt flakes is probably the easiest way to make every meal a gourmet one.

Penny buns are easy to find if you know their preferred habitat, for which it is useful to have some background tree knowledge: they are a type of ectomycorrhizal fungi, which forms underground relationships with trees, some of their favourites including beech, birch, oak, pine, fir and spruce. With a short but dramatic season, you can usually find penny buns a week or two after a heavy rainfall in early August until early October. *Amanita* mushrooms growing nearby are a good sign you're in the right kind of habitat.

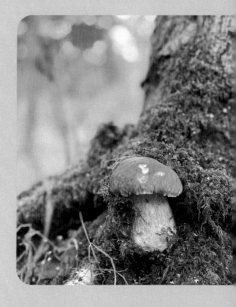

LOOKALIKES: **Summer penny bun (***Boletus reticulatus***), bay bolete (***Imleria badia***), bitter bolete (***Tylopilus felleus***)**

HARVEST TIME
Aug to Sept
FAMILY
Boletaceae
COMMON NAMES
Porcini, cep, king bolete, piggy
SPORE PRINT
Dark olive-brown

September

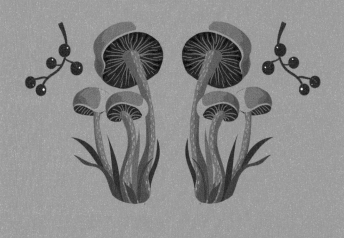

Out in the grasslands, morning dew settles on the orb webs made between the swathes of rosebay willow-herb, transforming each and every delicate strand into a glistening string of tiny pearls. St John's wort, yellow rattle and fleabane are all in bloom with their golden hues, and the changing leaves of rowan, guelder rose and hornbeam are now ablaze with colours of russet, copper and crimson, flickering like flames and casting a warm glow across the landscape.

In the woodlands, the mycelial strands that have laid dormant all year are now pushing up an abundance of mushrooms; decayers such as the puffballs, charcoal burners and deceivers hide among the leaf litter; a mass of parasitic honey fungus clumps around the base of a hollow beech; and chubby penny buns, scaly *Leccinums* and blushing *Amanitas* rest beneath a stand of knobbly birch trees like old friends.

The hedgerows are also an endless source of wonder in autumn – black and white bryony, dusty sloes and bright red barberries. These hedgerows, integral to our natural heritage, face continual threat, and regrettably, a significant number have succumbed to destruction. There are a number of local community planting and clean-up initiatives to take part in while out foraging across the autumn and winter months.

Giant puffball
Calvatia gigantea

The giant puffball is probably the easiest mushroom for first-time foragers to identify as it's so unmistakable, even from a distance – no wonder they are thought to be the first ever footballs!

HARVEST TIME
June to Sept
FAMILY
Agaricaceae
COMMON NAME
Football fungus
SPORE PRINT
Yellow to
olive-brown

Caution
Discard any mushrooms with yellow or brown centres, as they are going to spore and are past being edible.

Giant puffballs are white and spongey, with smooth skin. Instead of gills or a stem, a filament connects it to the earth. Generally spherical, they do 'split' with age. They smell nice and mushroomy, and should be completely white inside.

Strips of the dried mushroom can be used for starting fires when camping, while fresh spongey strips can be used to stem bleeding. Calvacin (obtained from C. *gigantea*) is recognized as one of the first anti-tumour substances ever derived from a mushroom. The puffball has also been used medicinally to promote muscle regeneration, help relieve inflammation and as a functional food to reduce blood sugar levels and help prevent diabetes.

Giant puffballs are an incredible free food source containing all nine essential acids (and all but one of the non-essential acids), and with just one fruiting body being able to feed an entire table of diners. Often breaded and eaten like a German schnitzel, thin slices can replace pasta sheets in a lasagne, and thick ones can be sliced for gluten-free pizza bases.

Find these mushrooms in fields and meadows, on roadsides and in parks, from summer through to early autumn.

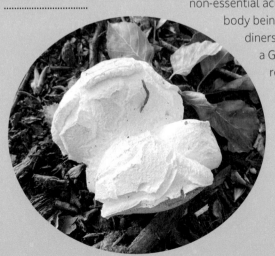

Beefsteak fungus
Fistulina hepatica

An interesting and somewhat creepy bracket mushroom that grows almost exclusively on oak trees in late summer through to late autumn – when sliced it looks eerily similar to raw meat!

As a polypore mushroom, beefsteak does not have gills but rather pores on the underside. Starting off as small pink blobs and eventually growing quite large, they flatten out to a 'shelf' before turning dark red and mushy. They are reddish-pink, tacky to the touch, marble just like fresh cuts of steak and even bleed a red liquid when cut.

The flavour is slightly citrusy, and the texture is more akin to watermelon than a sirloin. This is one of the few mushrooms that you can eat raw, and so it works well sliced thinly and served fresh as carpaccio, in salads, or marinated and dehydrated into plant-based jerky.

Oak seems to be their preferred habitat, but they are also found on sweet chestnut. Look for dying trees or those with injured limbs. They are best harvested once they have started to flatten out, while still firm to the touch.

HARVEST TIME
Sept and Oct
FAMILY
Fistulinaceae
COMMON NAME
Ox tongue
SPORE PRINT
Pinkish yellow

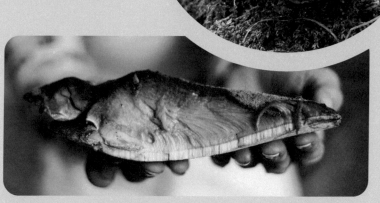

Hawthorn
Crataegus monogyna

HARVEST TIME
Apr to Nov
FAMILY
Rosaceae
COMMON NAMES
May tree,
mayflower,
thornapple,
hawberry,
whitethorn

An ancient tree steeped in folklore and an important host for hundreds of species of wildlife, the hawthorn has long been considered a staple source of food and medicine.

Grown as a hedge or as a tree that can reach over 10m (35ft) tall, hawthorn has shiny leaves divided into three to seven pairs of lobes. The leaves begin to emerge from the spiky branches in late March and are often in full leaf by late April. The sweet-smelling flowers have five petals that are white and often blushed with pink. In autumn, the thorny tree is laden with small, dark red fruits.

Hawthorn has been shown to increase the heart muscles' ability to contract, while also relaxing the blood vessels so that the heart both pumps better and has less resistance to pump against, raising low blood pressure and reducing high blood pressure. The berries are full of antioxidants and are typically prepared as a syrup or tincture for use as a heart tonic, an astringent, for muscle spasms and for high blood pressure and high cholesterol.

The leaves, flowers and fruits are all edible. The young spring leaves are medicinal as well as delicious, often described as being nutty in flavour or similar to that of apple skin. They can be added to salads, cooked as greens or dried and made into a tea. Flowers can be made into tea, tinctures, syrups and puddings, while the ripe berries have a soft, fibrous texture similar to avocado, and a slightly sweet flavour.

Flowers can be plucked from the tree when they appear in May; look for fresh, sweet-scented blossoms. Berries follow in autumn, when they can usually be found hanging from the trees.

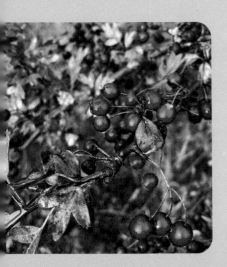

LOOKALIKE:
Blackthorn
(*Prunus spinosa*)

Hawthorn elixir

The quantities here depend solely on the size of jar used.

Hawthorn flowers
Ripe hawthorn berries
Haw-blossom brandy
Honey or sugar

1. Fill a clean jar halfway with ripe hawthorn berries.

2. Pour in the haw-blossom brandy to cover the berries.

3. Sweeten as desired with honey or sugar and leave to infuse for four to six weeks. Strain and bottle.

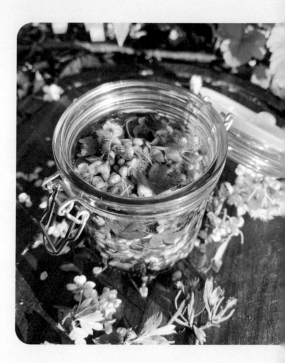

Suet pudding

550g (19½oz) shortcrust
   pastry
Handful of hawthorn
   buds
Chopped and cooked
   bacon, mushrooms
   and wild garlic

1. Roll out a pie crust long and thin.

2. Dot the crust with hawthorn buds, bacon, mushrooms and garlic.

3. Roll up, seal, and steam for an hour or two.

Common hazel

Corylus avellana

A deciduous tree, hazel is most commonly found in woodlands, where you will often find it is multi-stemmed as a result of coppicing. Look for trademark yellow catkins, the precursor to the delicious nuts.

HARVEST TIME
Year-round
FAMILY
Betulaceae
COMMON NAMES
Hazel, cobtree

If planted as a hedge, hazel can reach heights of 12m (40ft). The bark is shiny and has horizontal lines, or breathing pores, known as lenticels. The heart-shaped leaf has a serrated edge and the underside is covered in fine hairs. The male flowers are on long yellow catkins that droop down and release their edible pollen onto the tiny female flowers from December to April. Each flower bud develops into a cluster of hazelnuts with leafy bases, often called cobs.

Hazelnuts are an excellent source of protein and fatty acids. Blitz them into nut butter or a homemade hazelnut chocolate spread, soak them in water to make hazelnut milk, or crush and mix with sea salt and dehydrated penny bun for a crumb seasoning. Catkins, leaves and nuts can all be dried and ground into flour; catkins can be fermented and made into beer or soda; the bark can be made into a detoxifying tea to help treat colds.

Nuts are mature and ready to harvest in September and October, if the squirrels don't beat you to them first (see left)!

Beat the squirrels!
Harvest semi-green nuts straight from the tree in late September as long as they have started the ripening process, turning brown where they are attached to the husk.
Remove the husks and air-dry the nuts in single layers for good ventilation. Dry for a couple of weeks for long-term storage.

LOOKALIKES: **Lime tree (*Tilia* x *europaea*),
other *Lindens* (*Tilia*)**

Common beech
Fagus sylvatica

A deciduous tree with smooth, silver-grey bark and distinctive, toothed leaves with a hint of lemon, the beech tree is a common denizen of woodlands.

HARVEST TIME
All year-round
FAMILY
Fagaceae
COMMON NAME
European beech

These tall trees grow to 45m (150ft) or more, and have a domed crown and smooth, thin, grey bark. Young trees often have horizontal markings, whereas the bark on older trees becomes rough and starts to crack. Leaves are oval, have parallel veins and are pointed at the tip, with soft, silvery white hairs, and arranged alternately. When young the leaves are lime green, turning darker with age, and red and brown in autumn. Hard, prickly seed cases contain the edible beech nuts.

The oils in beech bark are thought to have insect-repellent qualities. The nuts, awesome toasted in a pan over the fire, are high in oil and protein. Young beech leaves are also edible, with a nutty flavour. They can be eaten fresh off the tree or added to salads, or made into a noyaux liqueur by steeping in gin for six to eight weeks, then making a sugar syrup, adding that alongside a splash of brandy and letting everything infuse in the dark for a month or so. Beech leaves help to clean the digestive system and stimulate the appetite.

Leaves appear in April and are best collected in the first couple of weeks while young and tender. Nuts are ripe and ready for harvest from September. These are easier to collect while on the tree, rather than trying to sift through the carpet of old casings from the previous year's drop. Placing the closed casings briefly over flames will help them to pop open.

LOOKALIKES: **Cultivated species of beech, including copper and purple varieties**

Caution
The nuts are tasty raw, but as with chestnuts, they have a high tannin content, so can cause an upset stomach if eaten in excess.

Fly agaric
Amanita muscaria

These are the mushrooms of folklore and fairy tale, of sacred drinks and ancient ceremonies. Though rarely deadly, they are potentially very toxic when eaten raw or improperly prepared.

HARVEST TIME
Sept and Oct
FAMILY
Amanitaceae
COMMON NAME
Fly amanita

Emerging from an 'egg sac', in less than a week this mushroom transforms into a large, unmistakable, cartoon-like mushroom with a bright red cap, still flecked with the white remnants of its universal veil, which are easily displaced by rain. The striated 'skirt', which was once covering the gills, drapes and hangs across the top of the white stipe in an elegant fashion.

Aside from their potent powers as an entheogen, *A. muscaria* have been eaten across the world for thousands of years, though proper preparation is crucial if you'd like to chow down on these mushrooms sans psychedelia. Boil the chopped mushrooms twice, each time for ten minutes; strain and use fresh water each boil. It is important to dispose of the spent cooking water, as accidentally drinking it could cause nausea or hallucinations. Afterwards, simply cook as you would with any other mushroom. If you don't feel comfortable preparing them for eating, a topical ointment or tincture can be made, which is said to be an effective treatment for sciatica, among other nerve pain issues.

Like all *Amanitas*, fly agarics are mycorrhizal, living symbiotically with certain trees, most often birch, beech and oak.

LOOKALIKES:
Red-coloured *Russula* spp.

Fly agaric topical tincture

Topical tinctures are a gateway to the wonderful world of medicinal mushrooms, and that of *A. muscaria* is said to be one of the most potent and effective of them all, providing instant relief to sciatica sufferers. Nature's very own ibuprofen!

If you create the double extraction detailed in step 4 below, it will keep well into the next mushroom season and beyond, and can be rubbed onto painful areas as and when needed, or you can soak a cloth in the liquid and use it as a compress.

Fly agaric mushrooms,
  to fill jar
High-proof alcohol
  (i.e. vodka)

Caution
DO NOT take this tincture internally: fresh A. muscaria *contain high levels of ibotenic acid and will likely make you sick. There are other methods for tinctures you can ingest, but this one isn't it.*

1. Fill a clean jar with the mushrooms and top with the alcohol.

2. Leave in a dark cupboard for four to six weeks and shake the jar every now and then.

3. Strain and decant.

4. Your alcohol extraction can be used as is, or you can create a double extraction for more potency: bring a pot of water to a simmer, add the mushrooms from the first extraction and simmer for a couple of hours, until around a 15 per cent reduction. Remove from the heat and let cool, then strain the mushrooms – the liquid is your water extraction. Add to the alcohol extraction to create a double extraction that is now shelf-stable.

Amethyst deceiver
Laccaria amethystina

HARVEST TIME
Aug to Nov
FAMILY
Hydnangiaceae
COMMON NAME
Amethyst laccaria
SPORE PRINT
White

A delightful little mushroom to spot, the brilliant purple colour makes them stand out against the leaf litter or moss of mixed woodlands. A variability in colour and shape is what gives them their common name of 'deceiver'.

Fairly small, usually around 2–8cm (1–3in) tall, amethyst deceivers are a vivid purple when young and wet, with purple flesh that dries out to a dull grey, almost white colour, in older mushrooms. The cap starts off convex and inverts as it matures, featuring widely spaced purple gills that are interspersed with shorter gills, and covered in a white spore print. Tough, fibrous stems are often twisted and contorted.

This is a mushroom that's often labelled as bland, or used just to add colour to plates, but I think they are lovely little mushrooms. I often gather these to fill out soups, stews and mushroom mixes in tarts and pastries.

Most commonly found in mixed woodlands – in great numbers – from late summer through to first frosts.

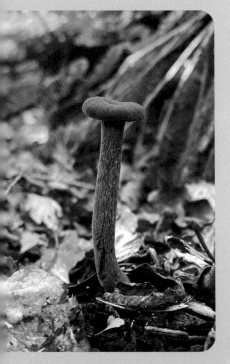

LOOKALIKES: ☠ Lilac fibrecap
(*Inocybe geophylla* var. *lilacina*),
☠ violet webcap (*Cortinarius violaceus*),
☠ lilac bonnet (*Mycena pura*),
common deceiver (*Laccaria laccata*)

Spear thistle
Cirsium vulgare

A tall, spiky biennial plant with distinctive globe-shaped purple flowers, most parts of spear thistle can be put to good use.

An erect plant reaching up to 1–1.5m (3–5ft), its long lanceolate leaves are rough, deeply lobed and tipped with large spines. The purple flowers are surrounded by spiky bracts and appear from June to October.

Traditionally an anti-inflammatory, spear thistle is used to treat arthritis and rheumatoid pains, and is also hailed as a diuretic and for treating digestive issues. Pickled spear thistle buds make a unique addition to salads or antipasto platters; experiment with different pickling spices for your own twist. Spear thistle also has a long, edible tap root that can be used much like burdock (see page 179).

Cook and eat young leaves and stems as spinach; leaves can be stripped of their stems and eaten, though it is the midrib of the leaf that is the most palatable, tasting like celery. Stalks can be stripped, chopped and added to stews, while the flower buds can be peeled and eaten like tiny artichokes, and pickled as a substitute for capers, though the effort (and pain!) rather outweighs the reward.

A common sight in meadows, fields, waste ground and roadside verges. Harvest the tap root in autumn, and young leaves and stems in spring or autumn. Store in the refrigerator for freshness or blanch and freeze for later use.

HARVEST TIME
Apr to Sept
FAMILY
Asteraceae
COMMON NAME
Bull thistle

....

Caution
Take care when harvesting as these are spiky plants, so don't forget your gloves!

....

LOOKALIKES:
**Creeping thistle
(*Cirsium arvense*),
marsh thistle
(*Cirsium palustre*)**

Sea buckthorn
Hippophae rhamnoides

HARVEST TIME
Sept to Mar
FAMILY
Elaeagnaceae
COMMON NAMES
Sea berry, sand
thorn, golden bush

A deciduous shrub known for its nutrient-rich orange berries, sea buckthorn contains bio-active substances and led to the development of radiation-protective creams for cosmonauts!

Sea buckthorn has narrow, lanceolate, silvery-green leaves in an alternate arrangement and often coated with silvery scales. Three-angled branches are armed with small, sharp thorns, helping the plant to form dense thickets. Yellow-green flowers are inconspicuous and appear in clusters along the spiked branches in spring. The most distinctive feature is its bright orange berries, which are small, round and densely packed.

A medicinal powerhouse containing many nutritional active compounds such as vitamins, fatty acids, phytosterols, polyphenols and carotenoids, the whole plant has been used

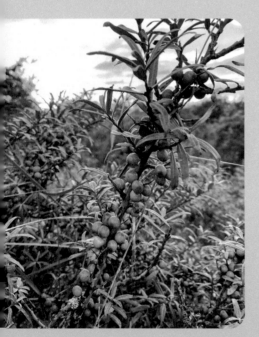

for medicine from the roots to the thorns, though it is the tart, citrusy berries that are reputed for their antioxidants and anti-inflammatory properties. The tangy berries are rich in vitamin C and can be used in jams, juices, sauces and desserts. The leaves can be brewed into a tea; alternatively, make a syrup by simmering berries with sugar and water.

Harvest ripe berries in late summer or autumn. Store in a cool, dry place or use immediately for culinary or medicinal purposes. Frequently found in coastal areas, sand dunes and dry, sandy soils, sea buckthorn is well adapted to withstand harsh conditions and is often planted to help combat soil and coastal erosion.

Crab apple
Malus sylvestris

The crab apple is an often underrated tree, with a tart fruit that is frequently seen hanging around on the branches well into autumn, and sometimes even early winter.

HARVEST TIME
May to Nov
FAMILY
Rosaceae
COMMON NAME
European wild
apple

With greyish-brown bark, mature trees have a lot of character, twisting and becoming knobbly as they age. The trees sport oval leaves with finely toothed serrated edges. White flowers form in late spring, and small, round, sour, yellow fruits in summer.

Crab apples are high in vitamin C. They are useful for maintaining gut health as they are also high in natural pectin, a prebiotic. This is the reason crab apples are often added to jams and jellies, as they help to provide a natural set. A tea made from the bark can help with insomnia and restless sleep. The tart flavour of the apples makes them a great addition to chutney, or a delicious butter that goes with just about anything. The fruit of cultivated trees found planted in streets or parks often vary in colour from yellow and green to red, giving a blushed colour to juice, sauces and syrups. Leftover skin, seeds and cores can be made into apple cider vinegar, and the acidity of crab apples makes them perfect for cider making.

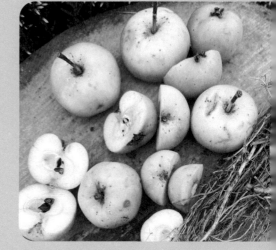

There are many varieties of crab apple, all of which are edible; however, the European native (*Malus sylvestris*) is threatened by hybridization from garden varieties, so it is always well worth noting and appreciating when you find one. Fruits are ripe when the seeds turn brown.

LOOKALIKES: **Other apple trees**

Crab apple &
wood avens whisky

Crab apples and wood avens give this whisky a warming spiced flavour. Use inexpensive whisky if you plan to sweeten it with sugar; if not, a smoother one would work better.

Made now, this tasty treat will be ready in time for Christmas gifting, however the longer you leave it to infuse the better – after a few years it will reach peak flavour, so try to make a couple of batches on your first go so you always have a bottle ready.

500g (1lb) crab apples
50g (2oz) wood avens
   roots
1 litre (2 pints) whisky
Optional: honey or sugar

The strained fruit can be added into cocktails, served alongside a cheeseboard, sliced and made into crab apple candies, cooked into a dessert sauce or baked into a boozy cake.

1. Halve the crab apples, roughly chop the wood avens root and place both in a large, sterilized glass jar.

2. Fill the jar with whisky, ensuring all the apples are submerged.

3. Let it sit for at least four to six weeks, allowing the alcohol to extract the colour and flavours from the apples and wood avens roots.

4. Strain out the fruit using a few layers of cheesecloth in a strainer.

Optional: Add sugar or honey to sweeten as desired, and let sit for a couple more days before decanting into bottles.

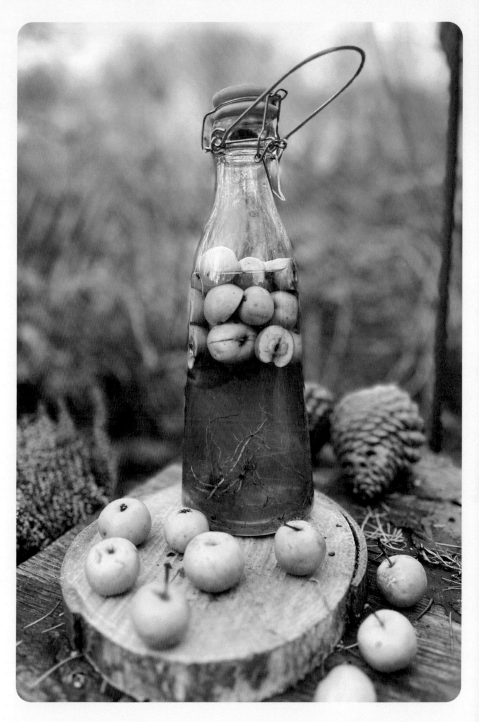

Cowberry

Vaccinium vitis-idaea

HARVEST TIME
June to Sept
FAMILY
Ericaceae
COMMON NAMES
Red whortleberry,
mountain
cranberry,
lingonberry,
foxberry

Tastier and much easier to harvest than cranberries, cowberries are used in much the same way, and have a delightful sometimes sweet but mostly sour flavour.

A low-growing, creeping, evergreen undershrub, cowberry's young leaves are tinged red and grow upright, whereas more established leaves are dark green and leathery, curled backwards, with a herringbone vein patterning, in-rolled margins and an alternate, or seemingly haphazard, leaf arrangement. Unopened flower buds are pinkish-red, opening up to drooping, bell-shaped flowers that have four out-curled white petals that are blushed with pink and huddle together in groups. Unripe fruits are green, turning to small, shiny bright red spherical berries clustered together on short upright stalks in autumn.

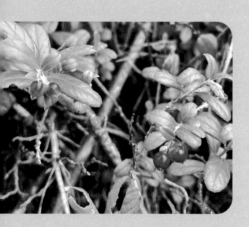

Containing vitamins A, B and C, as well as phosphorus, magnesium, calcium and potassium, cowberries can be frozen or dried for tea, cereal toppings and to be used in baking to boost the immune system, promote healthy gut bacteria and blood sugar levels, and reduce inflammation and risk of chronic disease, while also supporting heart, brain and eye health. Although some may find it too acidic to eat raw, once cooked down into jams, jellies, sauces and syrups, this super-fruit becomes sweet and delicious.

Cowberry can be found spread across large patches of moorland, heathland and acidic woodland, often growing alongside its close relative bilberry (see page 142). Berries start ripening in June, but often don't get going until early September. They contain benzoic acid, a natural preservative that will help keep them fresh in the fridge for up to a week.

LOOKALIKE:
Bilberry
(*Vaccinium
myrtillus*) before
fruiting

Parasol mushroom
Macrolepiota procera

Ants have a symbiotic relationship with these buff-coloured mushrooms, cultivating them to use as medicine, which is why you'll often find them near an ant hill.

HARVEST TIME
June to Oct
FAMILY
Agaricaceae
SPORE PRINT
Creamy white

Parasols form an egg shape initially, opening up to large flat mushroom roughly 30–40cm (12–16in) in diameter, and covered in scales appearing in rings across the cap, which stand 20–30cm (8–12in) high. They have fairly crowded, creamy white gills. The thin, creamy white, hollow stipe bears a brown snakeskin pattern and bulbous base, and the thick, fringed double skirt detaches.

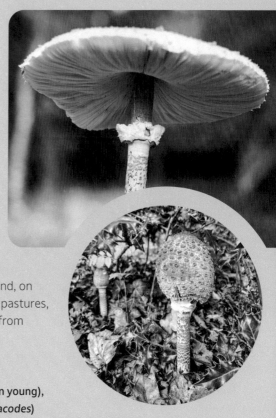

Parasols are delicious, with a rich, mushroomy, slightly sweet flavour, and their large size makes them a popular mushroom for soup, and also breaded into a schnitzel or escalope. Not just tasty, parasols also exhibit antibacterial, antioxidant, anti-inflammatory, antidepressant and anticancer effects.

This is a saprobic mushroom feeding off decaying organic matter, and they are found in woodland, on trails, in grassy clearings, glades and pastures, in troops, arcs and sometimes rings, from June to October.

LOOKALIKES: *Amanita* species (when young), shaggy parasol (*Chlorophyllum rhacodes*)

Hop
Humulus lupulus

HARVEST TIME
Aug to Oct
FAMILY
Cannabaceae

Hops are climbing plants with distinctive hanging cones, used in the production of beer.

Deeply divided leaves of three to five lobes with sharply serrated edges grow in an opposite arrangement on a twining vine, known as a bine. Cone-like structures called strobiles contain the hop flowers.

The flowers contain lupulin, a resin that contributes to beer's bitterness and aroma. Hop strains can vary drastically in flavour and can range from citrusy to garlicky, fruity, wheaty or sour. If you're not much of a beer drinker, try wilting the hops and eating as a green, infusing into oil or vinegar, adding to stews and soups, or making a digestive bitter to take before a meal or use in a cocktail. Utilize the sedative properties by making a stress-relieving tea to help treat restlessness, insomnia and excitability; you could even fill a calming herb pocket with hops to slip under your pillow for a blissful night's sleep.

Hop typically flowers between July and September and is usually ready to harvest between late August to early October. Test for ripeness by plucking a cone from the bine and giving it a squeeze – it should feel light and spring back to shape. Harvest your hops too early and you'll miss out on those complex bitter aromas. Where possible, harvest on the day you plan to use them. Find hop climbing through hedgerows, trees and bushes in meadow and along riverbanks and railway tracks.

LOOKALIKE: ☠ White bryony (*Bryonia dioica*)

Saffron milk cap
Lactarius deliciosus

This is perhaps the most highly sought after of milk caps. Why? The clue is in the Latin name, *deliciosus*! Its orange 'milk' is an important identifying feature and can be used to colour and flavour sauces.

The bright orange, pinkish cap is convex with an in-rolled margin when young, flattening and becoming vase-shaped when mature, forming a large central depression with blue green bruising. Caps can reach 6–20cm (2–8in) across, and the surface is often sticky when damp. The inside flesh has a fruity aroma and is firm and orange, with white or paler orange flesh nearer the centre. The crowded, shortly decurrent orange gills exude a peppery saffron-coloured 'milk' when cut or broken, which turns green once dried. The stipe is 5–8cm (2–3in) and the same colour as the cap, often tapering towards the base, sometimes having shallow pitting or darker spots on the upper.

Saffron milk caps are a rich source of beta-carotene, which is converted into vitamin A in the body and helps to maintain healthy organ functioning. They contain B-vitamins, including B2 (riboflavin) and B3 (niacin), minerals such as potassium and phosphorus, as well as antioxidants that help neutralize free radicals in the body, reducing oxidative stress and contributing to general health.

These fungi have a grainy, crunchy feel and a nutty flavour. The firm texture makes them ideal for pickling: clean and slice; prepare a pickling solution; blanch briefly; immerse in the solution; marinate for a few days.

Prefers acidic soils and is found in coniferous and mixed woodlands, forming mycorrhizal associations with pine and spruce trees (see page 40). Look for these mushrooms after a good rainfall.

HARVEST TIME
Aug to Nov
FAMILY
Russulaceae
COMMON NAMES
Delicious milk cap, red pine mushroom
SPORE PRINT
Cream to pale yellow

When gently pressed, the cap and stem should feel firm – avoid specimens that appear soft, as they might be past their prime.

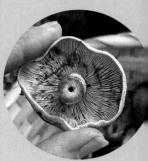

LOOKALIKES: **False saffron milk cap (*Lactarius deterrimus*), 💀 wooly milk cap (*Lactarius torminosus*)**

October

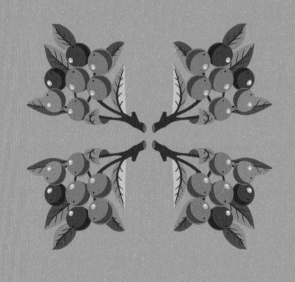

October is a month inoculated with wonder. Inside the mossy garden of the forest, glowing porcelain mushrooms feed from a decaying stump, their bright white gills reflecting up from the small pool of water that has gathered in the tree roots, and a group of black flies are hovering around a disturbed patch of ground under a hazel tree, indicating that truffles may be lurking just beneath the soil.

Beefsteak mushrooms give oak trees even more character this time of year, if that is at all possible, with their dark red fruiting bodies appearing like big floppy tongues poking out from wounds in the tree bark. The overpowering whiff of stinkhorn mushrooms is carried through the breeze, a curious fungus that I love to present on foraging forays – carving out the crunchy centre core and passing it round to guests for tasting often elicits a range of reactions!

The evenings are fading fast and the woodlands become a dark place on a grey day. Out in the fields, the lesser-seen waxcaps are starting to appear, putting on a spectacular display of colour. The hedgerows are still bursting with fruits, and the wild hops that have been scrambling through them all summer are now ready to harvest.

Blackthorn

Prunus spinosa

HARVEST TIME
Mar to Dec
FAMILY
Rosaceae
COMMON NAME
Sloe

Blackthorn is a thorny shrub with twisting branches, known for its bitter berries rich in vitamin C, which are commonly used to flavour spirits, with sloe gin being a popular festive drink at Christmas.

The rough, dark grey bark is bright orange inside, which peeks out when the surface is damaged or cut. Flowers have small, pretty white flowers with five petals, either singularly arranged or in pairs on the stems, appearing in March and April before the leaves. The dark leaves are small, slender and oval, but wider at the tip, with slightly hairy undersides and often tacky to the touch. The round fruits, or 'drupes', are called sloes or sloe berries. At around 1–2cm (¼–¾in), they are bluish-black with a whiteish 'bloom', or coating. Inside you will find one large stone and very bitter and astringent flesh.

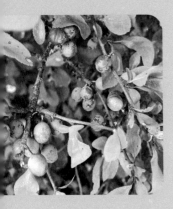

As an astringent, sloe berries can stimulate the metabolism, aid digestion and clear the body from toxins. The cooled tea made from steeping the leaves in hot water can be used as a mouthwash, gargled to help treat throat problems, or used as a soothing eye wash. The bark can also be powdered and made into a tincture to treat anxiety. The flowers can be made into almond-flavoured syrups, a blood cleansing tea or applied directly to the skin to ease rashes, while the leaves can be made into an aperitif.

Blackthorn makes for an almost impenetrable hedge when planted closely together. It is usually grown alongside the equally spiky hawthorn (*Crataegus monogyna*) and gorse (*Ulex*) as natural fencing and a wind barrier. Blackthorn is also planted in parks and in towns and cities for its early blossom. The berries sweeten slightly after a frost. Flowers appear early in March; leaves appear from April; sloes from late September through winter.

LOOKALIKES:
Cherry plum
(*Prunus*
***cerasifera*),**
hawthorn
(*Crataegus*
***monogyna*)**

Blackthorn leaf aperitif

Your aperitif is ready straight away but gets better with age! Drink as it is before a meal to stimulate the appetite, or pour over ice and add tonic or lemonade.

3 big handfuls of
    blackthorn shoots
    and leaves
300ml (10fl oz) gin
150g (5oz) sugar
1.5l (2½ pints) red or
    pink wine

1. Mix the ingredients together in a large container and give it all a good stir.

2. Cover and leave somewhere cool for two to three weeks, stirring every few days.

3. Strain the leaves and decant into a bottle.

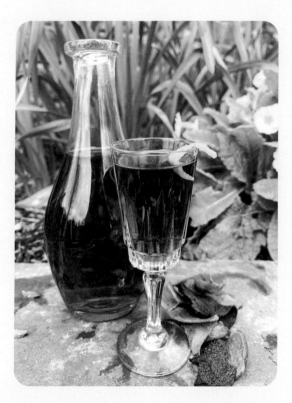

Common oak

Quercus robur

HARVEST TIME
Apr to Dec
FAMILY
Fagaceae
COMMON NAMES
English oak,
pedunculate oak

Reaching up to 40m (130ft) tall, some oaks are thought to be over a thousand years old. The acorns can be leached, dried and ground into flour, but did you know that the leaves are edible and medicinal too?

The leaf has a very short stalk, hidden by two small leaves, known as ears, at the base of each leaf. The acorns sit on the end of a long stalk called a peduncle.

A tea from oak leaves can be made to help fight inflammation, relieve colds and treat diarrhoea, and they can also be fermented with sugar, yeast, sultanas and a bit of ginger to make oak leaf wine. Oak leaves are also antiseptic and can be used directly on the skin as a styptic to help stem bleeding. Acorns are an abundant source of starch and fat, and can be used to make oil, soup, coffee, gluten-free flour or porridge, and I've even seen recipes for lacto-fermented acorn 'cheese' (though I am yet to try it out myself!).

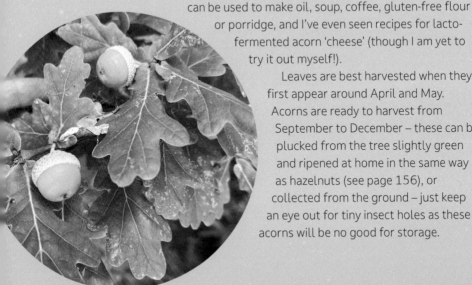

Leaves are best harvested when they first appear around April and May. Acorns are ready to harvest from September to December – these can be plucked from the tree slightly green and ripened at home in the same way as hazelnuts (see page 156), or collected from the ground – just keep an eye out for tiny insect holes as these acorns will be no good for storage.

LOOKALIKES: Holm oak (*Quercus ilex*), cork oak (*Quercus suber*), turkey oak (*Quercus cerris*)

Shaggy inkcap
Coprinus comatus

Not one to leave in your jacket pocket once harvested, the elongated egg-shaped shaggy inkcap – abundant in October – offers up not only a tasty mushroom, but also an edible ink.

HARVEST TIME
Aug to Nov
FAMILY
Agaricaceae
COMMON NAMES
Shaggy man, lawyer's wig
SPORE PRINT
Dark brown to black

The shaggy inkcap first peeks from the grass as a white, egg-shaped cap covered in shaggy scales, gradually opening up into the shape of a bell. The gills are crowded; first white, then pink and eventually turning black. The cap starts to liquefy from the margin until it almost entirely disintegrates. The tall white stipe is smooth, with a ring, or skirt, that can be easily displaced.

This is a delicious mushroom with a mild flavour, often used in creamy mushroom sauces. Look for them in grasslands, pastures, parks, fields and roadside verges, often in small groups. When harvesting, be sure to use the mushrooms in a timely manner – any delay and you will end up with a black mess! Young mushrooms still in their egg shape may keep refrigerated for a couple of days; however, be sure to place them in a bowl or container rather than a paper bag, as these mushrooms auto-digest in a process called deliquescence.

Luckily, the jet black ink is edible and can be stirred into pasta or preserved in butter. It can even be used as a natural drawing ink simply by mixing in a teaspoon of salt to act as a binding agent, prevent bacteria from growing and make your ink last longer.

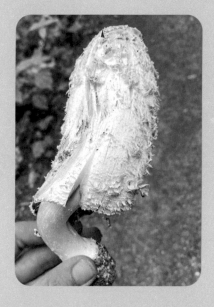

LOOKALIKES: Snowy inkcap (*Coprinopsis nivea*), magpie inkcap (*Coprinopsis picacea*)

Winter chanterelle
Craterellus tubaeformis

HARVEST TIME
Sept to Dec
FAMILY
Cantharellaceae
COMMON NAMES
**Trumpet
chanterelle, yellow
foot, yellow leg**
SPORE PRINT
Off-white

With its bright yellow legs, you'd be forgiven for thinking this mushroom would be an easy spot, but the brown trumpet cap makes it surprisingly sneaky, camouflaging among fallen autumn leaves. Still, it is worth the search, as winter chanterelle is very tasty.

The hollow, bright yellow stipes of these chanterelles are often grooved, appearing as two legs. The thin, funnel-shaped brown cap is often depressed in the centre, and has a wavy, undulating edge in older specimens. The gills are actually false gills and they appear as wrinkles or folds, with crossed veins beneath the cap surface. The mushrooms have a white to pale yellow spore print and a slightly sweet smell.

Winter chanterelles are excellent dried and pickled, their mild flavour lending well to both sweet and savoury dishes. As a mycorrhizal mushroom, you can find winter chanterelles carpeting the ground beneath certain trees – particularly pine, fir, spruce and beech – throughout autumn and winter. Chanterelles love moss, a water source and a slightly acidic environment. A prolific mushroom in good seasons, if you find a bounteous patch, you'll have chanterelles for years to come.

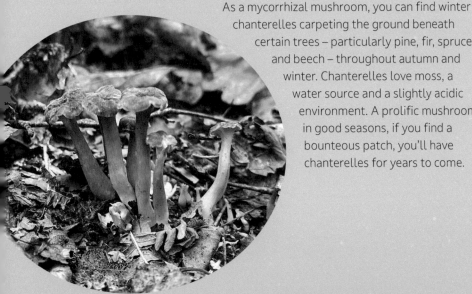

LOOKALIKES: **Jelly baby mushroom** (*Leotia lubrica*), **chanterelle** (*Cantharellus cibarius*)

Birch polypore
Piptoporus betulinus

A common bracket fungus growing exclusively on birch trees, *Piptoporus betulinus* is best known for its potent immune-boosting properties.

Easy to recognize by its semi-circular, white to tan-brown cap growing directly from the birch tree; when young, birch polypore can look like smooth, squashed golf balls emerging from cracks in the trunk. These start to colour and flatten out into a rounded shelf-like structure. This mushroom has tiny white pores on the underside rather than gills.

While edible, birch polypore is not typically consumed as a food due to its bitter taste and tough, woody texture. Instead, it is revered for its antibacterial, antiviral, antiparasitic and anti-inflammatory properties, most often prepared into immune-boosting teas and tinctures, or as a stock, soup or broth. For an anti-inflammatory, self-sealing plaster to help stem bleeding and prevent infection, score a rectangular shape into the underside and peel it off. When dried, birch polypore makes a great tinder, its smoke helping to deter insects.

When harvesting, look for young, firm, plump specimens with a clean, white underside. Use fresh, or store by drying or freezing. When preparing, simmer your mushrooms for at least an hour to extract the beneficial compounds and reduce bitterness. Common wherever birch trees reside, find them in particular on dead, dying, diseased or damaged trees.

HARVEST TIME	All year-round
FAMILY	Fomitopsidaceae
COMMON NAME	Razor strop fungus
SPORE PRINT	White

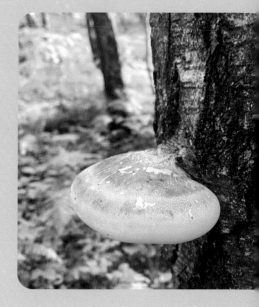

LOOKALIKE: **Artist's conk (*Ganoderma applanatum*)**

Bay bolete
Imleria badia

Looking similar to penny buns (and just as tasty!) is the bay bolete. The smooth, mat, chestnut brown cap can look velvety when dry, and viscid when wet.

HARVEST TIME
Aug to Nov
FAMILY
Boletaceae
SPORE PRINT
Olive-brown

Growing 5–15cm (2–6in) in height, with a cap diameter reaching 20cm (8in), the angular pores are pale yellow, turning lemon yellow with age and, more often than not, bruising to a deep blue when handled. The cap starts convex and flattens a little on older, larger mushrooms. The flesh is off-white, turning slightly blue around the tubes when cut, often with a deep red flush of colour just beneath the cap surface. A good identifying feature is its stipe: vertically lined markings with shallow brown ridges on a paler stem, usually with a slight curve to the base.

They can be used in much the same way as the penny bun (see page 149); I love to dehydrate them and keep them in jars in the pantry, pickle them in vinegar and spices, or preserve them in oil or salt for year-round umami flavour.

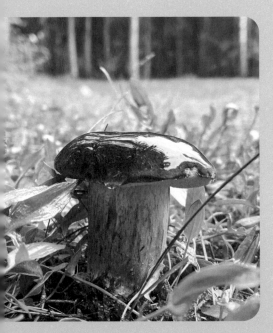

Boletes will have the texture of a soft sponge when past their best, so should be harvested when still firm to the touch. Find them under spruce pine, oak, beech and chestnut trees in late summer all the way through autumn. What's great about bay boletes is that they are usually maggot free, even when mature.

LOOKALIKES:
Brown birch bolete (*Leccinum scabrum*),
penny bun (*Boletus edulis*)

Burdock
Arctium

Burdock has heart-shaped leaves and pinky-purple flowers, with a root known for its starchy potato texture and delicious flavour similar to artichoke.

Burdocks are tall biennials, reaching 1.5–2.75m (5–9ft) at maturity. In the second year of growth, pink to purplish tufted flowers emerge, maturing into the familiar brown burs.

Medicinally, burdock is valued as a detoxifier, blood purifier, digestive aid and blood sugar regulator, as well as helping to treat inflammatory conditions such as rheumatism, psoriasis, eczema and other skin issues. The root is central for medicinal use, but leaves and seeds offer similar benefits and can be eaten, boiled for tea, steeped in alcohol for tinctures, or simply crushed and applied as a poultice.

Large leaves can serve as alternatives to tin foil or baking paper, and the flowers, equipped with hook-like spikes, have other practical uses, such as a makeshift button holder, and were thought to have been the inspiration for Velcro.

The root is the best-known edible part. For root harvesting, choose first-year plants with basal rosettes or second-year ones before flower stalks appear, for optimal tenderness. Flower stalks can be peeled and cooked, and bitter leaves and stems can enhance dishes while stimulating the digestive tract.

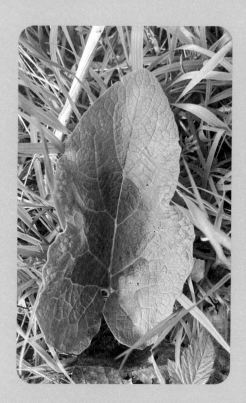

HARVEST TIME
Oct to Apr
FAMILY
Asteraceae
COMMON NAMES
Beggars burrows, thorny burr, button burr, cuckoo button

LOOKALIKE:
Milk thistle (*Silybum marianum*)

Hedgehog mushroom
Hydnum repandum

HARVEST TIME
Aug to Dec
FAMILY
Hydnaceae
COMMON NAME
Sweet tooth
SPORE PRINT
White

This mushroom is one of the safest to harvest for those new to foraging due to the distinctive 'teeth' on the underside of the cap.

A fairly stout mushroom with an irregularly shaped suede-like cap between 4–15cm (1½in–6in) in diameter, with decurrent spines that are off-white to apricot in colour and grow to around 5mm (⅛in) long. White stipe is firm, with off-white flesh.

Hedgehog mushrooms are high in calcium, iron, copper and magnesium, and have been shown to have antibiotic and anti-tumour effects. They have a sweet or nutty flavour and pleasant mushroomy aroma. The firm texture lends itself well to all types of cooking and storing, particularly pickles and ferments.

Long spines can make a mess and are often scraped from the underside of the caps before cooking – do this on-site when harvesting to help the mushrooms spread, or at least provide some food for woodland critters. Grows in troops or rings in deciduous woodland.

LOOKALIKE: **Terracotta hedgehog mushroom (*Hydnum rufescens*)**

Hen of the woods
Grifola frondosa

Cultivated as Maitake in Japan, China and Korea, hen of the woods grow in large clusters at the base of hardwood trees, particularly oaks, and have a rich umami flavour and a firm, meaty texture.

HARVEST TIME
Feb to Oct
FAMILY
Meripilaceae
COMMON NAMES
Lamb's quarters,
wild spinach,
goosefoot

The fruiting body is a large, multi-branched structure, with the individual branches, or fronds, growing in overlapping layers of rosettes with frilled edges, resembling a hen sitting in a nest. The mushroom is attached directly to the base of the tree from a short, central stipe. Hen of the woods can reach substantial sizes, with a diameter commonly reaching 1m (3ft). The colour ranges from pale to dark brown, and the underside is covered in fine, white pores. The flesh inside has an earthy, woody aroma, is white and does not stain black upon cutting.

Containing potent anti-tumour polysaccharides, in Chinese medicine extracts are used to inhibit tumour growth, metastasis and carcinogenesis. Hen of the woods has also been shown to treat palsy, nerve pain and arthritis, improve gut health and regulate blood sugar.

Prepare by sautéing or roasting, or add to soups and stews. These fungi contain proteolytic enzymes, which can help to tenderize meat. As they get so huge, you'll likely want to preserve them: dehydrate, pickle, freeze (cook first to prevent sogginess), or try making a jerky by thinly slicing, marinating and dehydrating.

Best harvested when the flesh is still soft and spongey. However, avoid harvesting the smaller 'baby' mushrooms – patience pays off, and later in the season you will be glad you waited. Found in both deciduous and mixed forests, and gardens.

LOOKALIKE:
Blackening polypore (*Meripilus giganteus*)

November

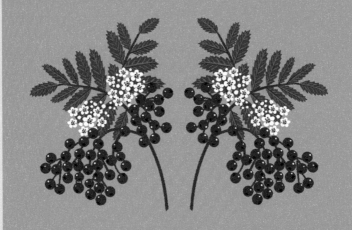

The weather is wild with gales, cold fog hangs in the air and the forest floor is crunchy underfoot. Jelly ear and birch polypores, the stalwarts of the woodlands, are once again joined by velvet shanks, but now the winter chanterelles, wood blewits and trooping funnels are also making an appearance, offering a last-minute chance to stock the pantry for the coming months.

In the fields and along the riverbanks, the dried seeds of dock, common hogweed, plantain and spear thistle sit atop their wiry stems, being gradually pecked off by hungry goldfinch. Rosehips and sorbus berries have ripened now that they have been kissed by frost, the purée-like flesh easily squeezed from the wrinkled skin, giving an unusually tropical flavour for this time of year.

While there is less wild food at its peak, November is still a fairly abundant month, with leafy greens such as sorrel, chickweed and bittercress to be found, but it's the roots that will now be of interest, as plants redirect energy downwards from their foliage. The roots and tubers of hedge garlic, mallow, nettle, cattail, horseradish, chicory, bistort, sweet cicely, water mint and meadowsweet can all be gathered this month.

Turkey tail

Trametes versicolor

HARVEST TIME
All year-round
FAMILY
Polyporaceae
COMMON NAMES
Rainbow fungus,
many-zoned
polypore
SPORE PRINT
White

Renowned for its vibrant hues and immune-boosting qualities, the turkey tail mushroom stands out in the world of medicinal Basidiomycetes. Flourishing predominantly on deceased hardwood, particularly oak and beech, this bracket fungus showcases concentric rings reminiscent of a turkey's tail.

This slender bracket fungus boasts a fan-shaped profile with multicoloured concentric rings akin to the plumage of a turkey. Its upper surface, slightly velvety and devoid of gills, reveals minuscule white to creamy-white pores beneath.

While non-toxic, turkey tail seldom graces the kitchen due to its formidable texture. Steeped in traditional medicine, its polysaccharopeptide richness hints at potent immune-boosting properties, and it has been used in decoctions or tinctures to fortify a weakened immune system. Simmered into a medicinal broth, it becomes a stalwart ally against chest infections and influenza.

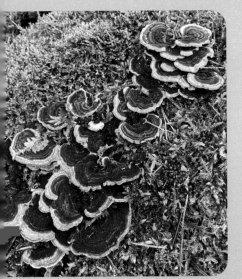

Widespread in woodland, parkland, hedges, gardens and anywhere trees and woody shrubs thrive, find it growing in tight clusters on small branches, fallen trunks and even park benches. Should the tiered structures of turkey tail grace a tree stump, the mushroom may adopt a rosette configuration. Harvest during the peak of autumn and winter, or year-round for diligent seekers. Seek out young, vivid specimens, steering clear of aged or deteriorating ones.

LOOKALIKE: **False turkey tail**
(*Stereum ostrea*)

Rowan
Sorbus aucuparia

A sacred tree in Celtic folklore, the buds and subsequent berries of the rowan are edible and highly beneficial – even the wood is strong and flexible, making it ideal for bushcraft.

HARVEST TIME
Apr to Nov
FAMILY
Rosaceae
COMMON NAMES
Luis, caorunn, mountain ash

Young rowans have a smooth, greyish-brown bark, which becomes rough and fissured with age, and they can grow up to 15m (50ft) tall. Leaves are dark green, fern-like and pinnate, with five to seven pairs of serrated leaflets and a single terminal leaflet. They turn red before falling in late autumn. Clusters of sticky buds appear in spring and open up to creamy white and heavily scented flowers, before ripening to bright red or orange berries, much like tiny apples.

Berries are high in vitamins (A and C), minerals (iron, potassium and magnesium), carotenoids, phenolic acids and pectin, and so boost the immune system and contribute to a healthy gut. The berries are quite astringent but sweeten after a frost, and make a delicious sauce or jelly that serves as a digestive aid for fatty foods. The buds have a sweet almond and/ or marzipan flavour and make a delicious syrup – add a handful to a pan with twice the volume of water, along with twice the volume of sugar, and simmer until the sugar is dissolved (do not let it come to a boil as this will alter the flavour).

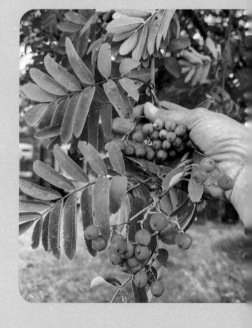

While rowan prefers a mountainous habitat, you can often find it in parks, on roadsides and in car parks. Berries start turning colour in late summer, and are usually ready to harvest in late autumn.

LOOKALIKES: **Other *Sorbus* spp.**

Snowy waxcap
Hygrocybe virginea

A small, delicate, ivory-coloured mushroom with a distinctive waxy appearance, the snowy waxcap is often found in grassy areas and woodlands in late autumn and early winter.

HARVEST TIME
Nov to Dec
FAMILY
Hygrophoraceae
SPORE PRINT
White

One of the easier waxcaps to identify by its snowy white cap of between 2–6cm (¾–2in), this mushroom is smooth in texture and has a conical shape. It often has a translucent character, especially when wet. Gills are thick, fleshy, widely spaced and decurrent; the stipe is white and cylindrical, often appearing off-white or grey at the base; the spore print is white.

Snowy wax caps are tasty little mushrooms that can be found speckled across fields at a time when it's slim pickings for many other fungi. Try them pan fried in butter or add to pickling jars. Frequently found in grassy areas, meadows, playing fields and woodlands, either singularly or in small clusters, snowy waxcaps can be prolific in number due to being able to tolerate a higher soil fertility, enabling the mushroom to recolonize an area more quickly than other waxcap species. Though snowy waxcaps are the hardier of the waxcap bunch, they should be foraged only where abundant as, due to the over-application of harmful chemicals sprayed across our countryside, this mushroom's preferred habitat is becoming increasingly uncommon.

LOOKALIKES: **Meadow waxcap (*Cuphophyllus pratensis*),** ☠ **fool's funnel (*Clitocybe rivulosa*)**

Meadow waxcap
Cuphophyllus pratensis

Meadow waxcap is one of the largest and most common members of the waxcap family, gracing unimproved grasslands, upland pastures and acidic meadows during autumn and early winter.

HARVEST TIME
Oct to Jan
FAMILY
Hygrophoraceae
COMMON NAMES
Salmon waxy cap,
butter meadowcap
SPORE PRINT
Off-white

The meadow waxcap starts life with a domed, slightly umbonate cap gracefully flattening in form as it matures, with edges turning upwards and a size ranging between 2–8cm (¾–3in) across. Variable in colour from yellowy-orange to peach, it has a waxy appearance, although is dry to the touch, except in wet weather. The thick, fleshy, decurrent gills are broad, widely spaced and feature cross veins. The solid stout stem is a similar colour to the cap and becomes hollow with age.

Taking a bit longer to cook than many other mushrooms, due to their high water content waxcaps can be cooked in their own juices. Use the leftover cooking water for soups and stocks. Toss chunks into omelettes, breakfast wraps or a galette. The mild mushroomy flavour and firm flesh means they are great for pickling too.

Though a fairly abundant mushroom, waxcaps are becoming increasingly rare across Europe due to their sensitivity to fertilizers, pesticides and herbicides, and the subsequent loss of their preferred habitat. Therefore, meadow waxcaps should be gathered only where they are plentiful.

LOOKALIKE:
☠ Ivory funnel (*Clitocybe dealbata*)

Guelder rose

Viburnum opulus

HARVEST TIME
All year-round
FAMILY
Adoxaceae
COMMON NAMES
Water elder,
swamp elder,
cramp bark,
European
cranberry bush

The glossy, translucent red berries of the guelder rose ripen in summer and have an unpleasant, musky smell. While astringent and mildly toxic when raw, they are edible when cooked and are commonly used as a substitute for cranberries.

The guelder rose can reach heights of up to 4m (13ft) and can be distinguished easily from other trees by its maple-like leaves, which are dark green, opposite and palmately lobed, with three distinct lobes, serrated edges, deep veins and fine hairs on the underside. In late autumn, these leaves turn a vibrant copper red. Umbels of white flowers cover the tree in spring; the large sterile flowers around the outside are to entice pollinators to the smaller, fertile flowers on the inside of the umbel. The red berries, often referred to as 'drupes', hang in bunches and contain a hard seed.

The berries are a great source of vitamins A, C, E and K, as well as iron, manganese, calcium, potassium and phosphorus. An easy way to harness these powers is by making a syrup or tea, which will help to relieve indigestion, a sore throat and coughing. The smooth, pale, greenish-brown bark is known as 'cramp bark' and has been traditionally used as a muscle relaxant to help alleviate menstrual cramps and pain.

Guelder rose is often found along hedgerows, in scrub and near water sources, including streams and damp woodlands. Harvest berries when fully ripe, which is usually in late autumn. Inner bark and young twigs can be harvested all year-round.

LOOKALIKE: **Field maple (*Acer campestre*)**

Wood blewit
Clitocybe nuda

A cold-weather mushroom that can be identified by its stocky stature and violet to purple-blue cap, wood blewits are a sure sign that autumn is truly here.

Standing at around 5–10cm (2–4in) tall, wood blewits have caps 5–15cm (2–6in) in diameter. The stipe fades with age, and the gills always have a noticeably blue hue, even when mature.

These are delicious mushrooms with a rich flavour, faint aniseed smell and wonderful texture, especially when harvested while young and firm. They are high in dietary fibre and low in fat and sugar, while also boasting beta-glucans, offering anti-tumour, antioxidant, immunomodulation, anti-microbial, hypoglycaemic and cholesterol-lowering effects.

Wood blewits are a saprobic mushroom and feast on decaying wood or leaf litter. You can often find them in coniferous and broadleaf woodland, as well as in church grounds and park and field edges, often growing in rings, even well into frosty weather. For a reliable source, consider cultivating them at home.

HARVEST TIME
Oct to Jan
FAMILY
Tricholomataceae
COMMON NAMES
Blue hats,
blue foot
SPORE PRINT
Pale pink

LOOKALIKES:
☠ Violet webcap (*Cortinarius violaceus*), Sordid blewit (*Lepista sordida*), Field blewit (*Lepista personata*)

Caution
Take care when foraging for wood blewits as lookalikes include toxic species from the Cortinarius *genus, so stay away from any mushrooms with rust-coloured spores or deposits left on the stipe (or any with cobwebs attached to the gills).*

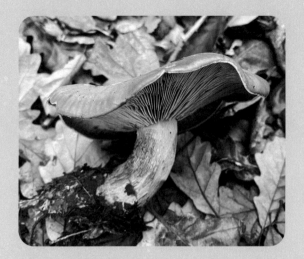

December

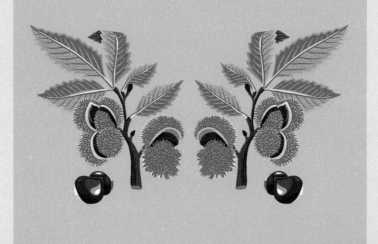

With the framework of the forest laid bare, winter is an opportunity to observe the way in which trees and shrubs grow, their buds, branching arrangements and overall shape becoming easier to determine without the distractions of fruit, flowers and the canopy of green.

The conifers start to take the spotlight, especially when dusted with a sprinkling of snow. Aside from the occasional winter mushroom, there is little still growing in the woodlands but vast stretches of ivy, and though inedible, a small basket of leaves can be gathered and boiled to make a natural washing detergent. The sharp thickets of holly and their glossy red berries provide natural materials for wreath and garland making in time for Yule, another gentle afternoon activity to make you feel as though you've had a productive forage.

By closely observing the shifting seasons and understanding the life cycles of plants and fungi, we cultivate an attunement to the natural rhythms of our surroundings. This heightened awareness not only allows us to appreciate the interconnectedness of all living things but also provides invaluable insights into their habitats and the optimal times for harvesting various plant and fungal species. This, in turn, ensures a foraging experience characterized by enhanced flavour, nutritional value, and a holistic, sustainable approach, fostering a more harmonious relationship with nature.

Common sorrel

Rumex acetosa

A perennial herb with a vibrant citrusy tang, sorrel is easily recognizable by its arrow-shaped leaves and red-tinged seed heads.

HARVEST TIME
All year-round
FAMILY
Polygonaceae

The bright green leaves have a pointed 'fish tail' with backwards-facing basal lobes. In late spring and early summer, the plant bears inconspicuous green flowers that turn red in the sun and appear on tall, ribbed stems.

Sorrel is rich in antioxidants, fibre and manganese, helping to regulate blood sugar levels and maintain heart and bone health. Its vitamin A content helps to maintain eyesight and skin, and it's also loaded with vitamin C, which means it can help to fight off inflammation and give your immune system a boost during the winter months.

The leaves are best eaten raw and harvested when young and tender, with a flavour akin to cooking apple peel. They can be used in salads and both sweet and savoury dishes. Sorrel makes a refreshing granita when made into a syrup and frozen. The citrusy taste is due to oxalic acid, a naturally occurring compound in many foods we commonly eat, such as spinach, kale and dark chocolate. Small amounts are safe but it should be eaten in moderation, as it can inhibit the absorption of important nutrients.

Widespread, sorrel is found year-round in grasslands, meadows and open areas, with a preference for well-drained, slightly acidic soil. It is more noticeable in winter, when grass is short.

LOOKALIKES: **Sheep's sorrel (*Rumex acetosella*), Wood sorrel (*Oxalis acetosella*), ☠ lords-and-ladies (*Arum maculatum*)**

Sea beet

Beta vulgaris subsp. *maritima*

A wild ancestor of cultivated beetroot, sugar beet and Swiss chard, sea beet is a coastal plant with tender, spinach-like leaves that can be eaten raw or cooked – but the flowers and stems are arguably the best parts.

HARVEST TIME
All year-round
FAMILY
Amaranthaceae
COMMON NAME
Wild spinach

Sprawling and clump forming in habit, sea beet is recognizable by its glossy, dark green, arrow-shaped leaves with deep veins, wrinkled margins and reddish stems. As the plant matures, the leaves become irregular and undulating, deepening in colour. Clusters of flowers adorn tall stems and appear from June to October.

A great source of iodine, sea beet helps to regulate hormones, metabolism and body temperature. It is said to be effective against intestinal tumours and helps to detoxify the body. The succulent and nutty leaves are available all year-round, but are sweeter and more tender when harvested young; older, more leathery leaves can be cooked as you would chard or spinach, and they make good protective wraps for food when cooking over a direct flame, helping to lock in flavour and moisture. Flowering stems can be steamed or sautéed as a side dish, or chopped into soups and stir fries.

Sea beet often grows in coastal areas, tolerating salty conditions such as cliffs, shingle beaches, salt marshes, esplanades and along sea walls.

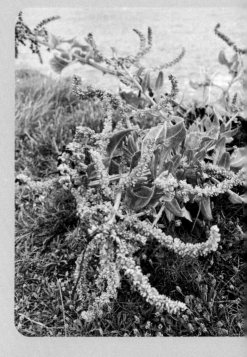

LOOKALIKES: **Other beet species, dock species, horseradish (*Armoracia rusticana*), sea kale (*Crambe maritima*)**

Mahonia
Mahonia aquifolium

An evergreen shrub with stiff holly-like leaves and clusters of small, bright yellow flowers, mahonia is valued for its ornamental and medicinal properties, and yellow spikes of sweet-smelling flowers.

HARVEST TIME
Nov to July
FAMILY
Berberidaceae
COMMON NAME
Oregon grape
holly

Growing up to 3m (10ft) tall, mahonia has a tiering habit with pinnately compound, spiny leaves. Clusters of small yellow flowers grow along erect spikes, or racemes, with flowers appearing in early winter all the way through until next spring.

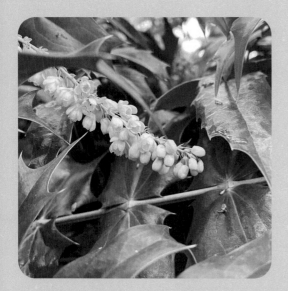

Mahonia is known for its berberine content, which has antimicrobial properties and helps to strengthen the heartbeat; it has also been helpful in treating digestive issues and skin conditions. The berries are much more nutritious that blueberries, and much higher in inflammation-fighting antioxidants, too.

Flowers can be eaten raw and have a sweet honey tang. In late summer or early autumn, they give way to dark blue, elongated grape-like berries that are tart and acidic, though these do sweeten after a few frosty nights. Berries can be eaten raw or used in jams, jellies or teas, fermented into wine, or even dried and used year-round for baking or as a cereal topper.

Mahonia is common in woodlands, hedgerows, gardens, parks and shaded areas.

Caution
Some people may experience stomach upset when digesting mahonia, so moderation is advised.

LOOKALIKE: 💀 Holly (*Ilex* spp.)

Sweet chestnut
Castanea sativa

A huge tree in maturity, the sweet chestnut bears delicious nuts synonymous with the winter festive season, and they are also great for the gut.

Reaching up to 35m (115ft) tall, the sweet chestnut sports a smooth grey bark often featuring long diagonal cracks or fissures. The leaves are long, glossy and oblong, with many pairs of prominent parallel veins, a pointed tip and a coarsely serrated edge. The green leaves turn orange, gold, then brown in autumn. Long, erect catkins appear in spring, replaced in autumn by green balls that have dense, flexible spines. Within each ball are two to four shiny brown nuts.

Sweet chestnuts are high in fibre, so help to aid digestion and prevent blood sugar spikes, and they're full of beneficial bacteria too. The only nuts that contain vitamin C, they're also high in antioxidants, helping to reduce cardiovascular issues and suppress chronic inflammation.

Use your foraged chestnuts to make a delicious purée or butter for sweet or savoury dishes. Grind them into flour, add them to your Christmas stuffing, or make glazed candied chestnuts for a sweet treat. The inner bark is great for tinder.

To make harvesting a less a painful affair, try using your feet to pry open the casing, and carefully grab the chestnut by the little tufts at the top of the nut. Usually one nut is larger than the others – these are the ones to gather.

HARVEST TIME
Oct to Dec
FAMILY
Fagaceae
COMMON NAME
Spanish chestnut

LOOKALIKE:
☠ Horse chestnut (*Aesculus hippocastanum*)

Chestnut & meadowsweet butter

There are so many layers of happiness to this recipe – rummaging through the crunchy leaves in search for the chestnuts, roasting them over a fire, the divine smell of the meadowsweet-infused milk, and lastly, the endless treats that could be made from it.

If you've already got a stash of roasted chestnuts waiting to be used up, you could be enjoying this butter within just half an hour! Use it on toast or in both sweet and savoury pastries, bake a chestnut cake, or make the traditional chestnut dessert, Mont Blanc.

1 tbsp honey or sugar
500ml (2 cups) milk
500g (1lb) roasted, peeled and chopped chestnuts
2 tbsp meadowsweet seeds

For a sweeter version, add chocolate chunks to the food processor.

1. In a saucepan over a medium heat, whisk together the honey or sugar with the milk (I love to use nutty-tasting hemp-seed milk, but you can use your favourite milk, or even water) until dissolved.

2. Add the chestnuts and meadowsweet seeds and simmer for 20 minutes, until it has reduced by half.

3. Sieve the mixture and save the milk to one side.

4. Transfer the nuts into a food processor and blend until smooth, adding the milk back in little by little until it reaches your desired consistency.

5. Store in the fridge for a few days, or portion it up and pop it in the freezer.

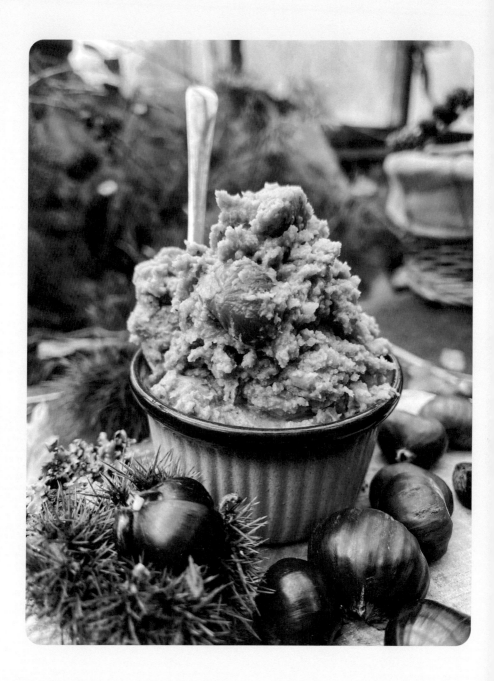

Winter cress

Barbarea vulgaris

This highly nutritious flowering wild green is a fairly tall, slender branching biennial plant.

HARVEST TIME
Nov to Jun
FAMILY
Brassicaceae
COMMON NAMES
Yellow rocket,
winter rocket

Glossy, dark green basal leaves are pinnate with two to five pairs of lateral lobes, with the terminal lobe having a rounded serration. Upper leaves are typically unlobed, and alternate on furrowed stems. Lower leaves can sometimes turn reddish in the summer. Hairless flower buds open up into small, vibrant yellow, four-petalled cruciform flowers on tight, terminal clusters, which develop into tough, narrow, erect seed pods 1–4cm (½–1½in) in length.

Leaves of winter cress can be used in the same way as spinach or collard greens; alternatively, mix raw leaves in with other salad greens to mask the slight bitterness. Flowers are delicious sautéed, or harvest the top few centimetres of the plant just before the buds burst open and eat them in favour of sprouting broccoli, which has just half the vitamin A of winter cress and less than a third of its vitamin C. The dried seeds can be used as a mustard seed substitute, containing the same healthy glucosinolates.

Often found sprawling along riverbanks and wet woodlands from November through to June.

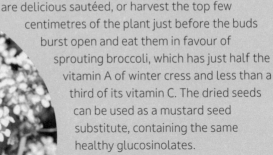

LOOKALIKE: **Watercress**
(*Nasturtium officinale*)

Horseradish
Armoracia rusticana

Horseradish has a long tap root where it not only stores most of its nutrients, but also most of its flavour.

A tall, long-lived perennial plant, horseradish often reaches 1m (3ft) in height, and has an upright, clumping habit. The large, elongated oblong leaves can grow up to 80cm (31in) in length and are dark green and glossy, with a wavy, undulating edge and prominent white central rib. When horseradish flowers it sends up small, simple white flowers with four petals.

Horseradish helps to aid digestion and speed up the metabolism. It is also antibacterial, and helps to boost the immune system and protect against cancer and brain disease, thanks to the minerals and glucosinolate plant compounds. It is used to clear the sinuses and relieve colds and blocked noses, and is an effective remedy for bronchitis. A compress of the leaves can be used to treat wounds and reduce scarring.

Horseradish sauce is made from the root, freshly grated and stirred into vinegar, salt and sugar. The root can be dried and ground into powder or sliced thinly and baked into crisps, while leaves can be chopped and added to salads and stir fries or mashed into potato. Use fresh, or freeze or dry for long-term storage. Leaves can be harvested all year; use them fresh, dried, or preserved in oil. The flowers make a spicy addition to salads, and the young stems can be chopped and cooked into meals or chomped on raw, if you dare!

Find it everywhere from waste grounds to field edges and meadows, and sometimes as garden escapees.

LOOKALIKE: **Dock species (*Rumex*)**

HARVEST TIME
All year-round
FAMILY
Brassicaceae
COMMON NAME
Red cole

Roots
If harvesting for roots, dig up in late autumn or winter, as a frost will improve the flavour.

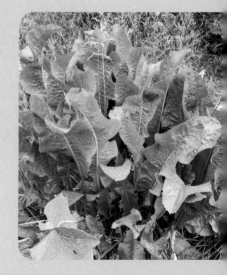

Wild ingredients

Here are some ways to utilize your harvest and incorporate wild foods into everyday meals, without necessarily replacing familiar ingredients.

Foraged garnishes Add a touch of wild beauty to your dishes with edible flowers, leaves or small fruits as garnishes. They can enhance the visual appeal of your meals and introduce unique flavours.

Infused oils and vinegars Create infused oils or vinegars by steeping wild herbs or flowers in olive oil or vinegar. Use to add a hint of wild flavour to salads, marinades and dressings.

Wild pesto Make wild pesto using foraged greens such as hedge garlic, nettles or wild ramps. Spread on bread, mix into pasta or use as a dip.

Pickled delights Experiment with pickling wild vegetables, such as burdock stems or young milkweed pods. Serve alongside main dishes or as tangy additions to charcuterie boards.

Fruit preserves Turn wild berries into jams, jellies or chutneys. Enjoy on toast, paired with cheese or use to glaze meats.

Wild smoothies Incorporate wild berries, greens or herbs into your morning smoothie for a nutritional boost and a taste of the wild.

Floral water Infuse water with the essence of edible flowers for a refreshing and aromatic beverage. Think of it as a homemade herbal spa water.

Wild-inspired baking Incorporate wild ingredients such as dried berries, nuts or seeds into baked goods, from cakes and cookies, to bread and crackers.

Wild alternatives to common herbs and spices

Allspice: Common hogweed seed
Almond: *Prunus* blossom and pits,
Sorbus young leaf and blossom
Aniseed: Wild fennel, sweet cicely,
aniseed agaric mushroom
(*Clitocybe odora*)
Caraway: Wild carrot seed
Cardamom: Common hogweed seed
Celery seed: Alexanders seed,
lovage seed
Chilli: Water pepper
Cinnamon: Wood avens root
Clove: Wood avens root
Coconut: Gorse flower,
blackberry buds
Coriander: Common hogweed, angelica
Cumin: Angelica seed
Curry leaf: Spignel, Himalayan
balsam seed
Dill: Wild fennel
Fenugreek: Lovage
Garlic: Ramsons, three-cornered leek
Ginger: Magnolia petals, sweet myrtle
Lemon: Lemon balm, sorrel, sumac,
young conifer needles
Pepper: Nasturtium, pepper dulce,
pepperweed, peppery bolete
mushroom (*Chalciporus piperatus*),
sneezewort
Rosemary: Ground ivy
Mustard: Sea rocket, sea radish,
scurvy grass, honesty seeds,
cuckooflower, charlock
Onion: Hedge garlic, crow garlic

Orange zest: Sea buckthorn
Oregano: Marjoram
Salt: Seaweeds
Vanilla: Meadowsweet, sweet
woodruff, lady's bedstraw

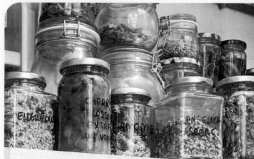
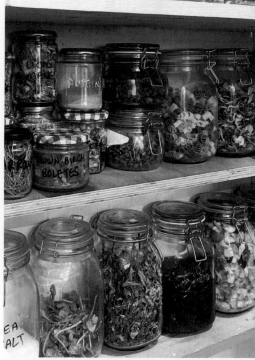

FORAGED FIRST AID KIT

Turning to nature to harvest its vast array of remedies is an age-old, trusted way to self-medicate for minor injuries and common everyday health complaints. Here are some herbal alternatives you can make to replace and/or enhance traditional items in a typical first aid kit. Remember to label each product clearly, including ingredients and usage instructions.

Also, keep in mind that while herbal remedies can offer gentle support for various situations, it is important to have a basic understanding of their properties and potential interactions. Consulting with a healthcare professional is advised, especially for serious injuries or health concerns.

HERBAL SALVE

Alternative to Antibiotic ointment.

To make Use infused oils (yarrow, plantain, sneezewort) and beeswax.

Applications Minor cuts, scrapes and burns.

HEADACHE TEA

Alternative to Headache tablets

To make Infuse roots such as dandelion, burdock and common dock in hot water, add a few drops of feverfew tincture to half a cup of tea and drink until symptoms subside.

Applications Vascular headaches and migraines.

THROAT SPRAY

Alternative to Antiseptic spray.

To make Infuse herbs such as mint, elderberry and mallow into water and add to a mister.

Applications Sore throats.

CHAMOMILE EYE WASH

Alternative to Eye-wash solution.

To make Fill small muslin bags with dried chamomile flowers.

Applications Irritated eyes.

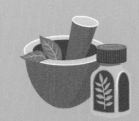

HERBAL COLD COMPRESS

Alternative to Cold packs.

To make Fill cloth bags with herbs such as chickweed, clover and fat hen, infuse into hot water and leave to cool. Place in the freezer for 15 minutes before applying.

Applications Minor injuries.

HONEY PASTILLES

Alternative to Cough sweets.

To make Combine finely powdered dried herbs and berries such as devil's bit scabious, guelder rose and sorrel with honey, roll into balls and refrigerate to harden. Suck, chew or dissolve in a drink.

Applications Coughs and colds.

MUGWORT CREAM

Alternative to Hydrocortisone creams.

To make Combine mugwort-infused oil and shea butter.

Applications Skin irritations.

STEAM INHALER

Alternative to Decongestant.

To make Fill a bowl with herbs such as marjoram pine and mullein, pour over boiling water, drape a towel over your head and position yourself over the bowl.

Applications Mild respiratory relief.

HERBAL GAUZE PADS

Alternative to Medical gauze pads.

To make Infuse sterile gauze pads with herbal infusions such as plantain or comfrey.

Applications Dressing wounds.

DIGESTIVE TEA BAGS

Alternative to Antacids.

To make Prepare herbal tea bags with soothing herbs such as hops, burdock and fennel.

Applications Digestive discomfort.

HERBAL RESCUE REMEDY

Alternative to Stress-relief products.

To make Create a tincture with calming herbs such as St John's wort, gorse and motherwort.

Applications Stress and anxiety.

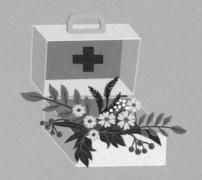

Index

Acknowledgements

Thanks to the ever patient Emily, Katie and Tokiko at Quercus, to Jo Parry for the beautiful, enchanting illustrations, to all of the ethnobotanical teachers and mycologists I have learnt from over the years – and still continue to learn from – and, of course, to Chris and Penny for their love and support.

Thanks to the following for images supplied:
p7 Introduction portrait – Joe Earley
p135 Chicken of the woods – Huenuman Coloma p153 Beefsteak (top image) – Christopher Price
p153 Beefsteak (bottom image) – Joe Earley
p161 Spear thistle – Sarah Emma Smith

iStock
19 Igor Kramar; 20 MortenChr; 23 Michel VIARD; 27 Werner Meidinger; 31 Mantonature, Tom Meaker; 65 Mantonature

Shutterstock
20 Jolanda Aalbers; 23 Isaenko, Gabriela Beres; 24 Rudenko Yevhen; 27 agatchen; 28 Alexey Kharin, Cyrustr; 31 Martin Fowler; 41 YevgeniyDr; 56 Iva Vagnerova; 78 Tomasz Czadowski; 92 Anastasiia Malinich; 93 Orest Iyzhechka; 94 Tom Meaker; 99 Brookgardener; 125 arousa; 130 Danny Hummel; 131 PaniYani; 133 Hana Stepanikova; 145 COULANGES; 157 footageclips; 168 guentermanaus; 181 Gertjan Hooijer; 198 ArgenLant

Wikimedia Commons
20 Andreas Kunze; 28 Alex Lockton

First published in Great Britain in 2024 by Greenfinch

An imprint of Quercus Editions Ltd
Carmelite House
50 Victoria Embankment
London EC4Y 0DZ

An Hachette UK company

A CIP catalogue record for this book is available from the British Library

HB ISBN 978-1-52943-712-6
Ebook ISBN 978-1-52943-713-3

10 9 8 7 6 5 4 3 2 1

Design by Tokiko Morishima
Illustrations by Jo Parry

Printed and bound in China

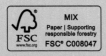

Papers used by Greenfinch are from well-managed forests and other responsible sources.